Staying SOBER

Staying SOBER

A Nutrition and Exercise Program for the Recovering Alcoholic

JUDY MYERS
with Maribeth Mellin

CONGDON & WEED, INC.
New York • Chicago

Library of Congress Cataloging-in-Publication Data

Myers, Judy.
  Staying sober.

  Bibliography: p.
  1. Alcoholics—Rehabilitation.   2. Alcoholism—
Nutritional aspects.   3. Alcoholism—Diet therapy.
4. Exercise therapy.   I. Mellin, Maribeth.   II. Title.
[DNLM: 1. Alcoholism—rehabilitation—popular works.
WM 274 M996s]
RC565.M94   1987   616.86'106   87-6881
ISBN 0-86553-172-2

Jacket photo by Michael Franchino.
Interior photos by John Balik, except photo on page viii by
Jonathan Prism Studios.

Epigraph on page 7 from column entitled "Nutrition Without
Charge" by Ann Landers, Los Angeles Times Syndicate.
Reprinted by permission.

Library of Congress Catalog Card Number: 87-6881
International Standard Book Number: 0-86553-172-2
                                    0-8092-0172-2Z (Contemporary
                                               Books, Inc.)
Published by Congdon & Weed, Inc.
A subsidiary of Contemporary Books, Inc.
298 Fifth Avenue, New York, New York 10001
Distributed by Contemporary Books, Inc.
180 North Michigan Avenue, Chicago, Illinois 60601

Published simultaneously in Canada by Beaverbooks, Ltd.
195 Allstate Parkway, Valleywood Business Park
Markham, Ontario L3R 4T8 Canada

*To all those people throughout the world
who want to recover from alcohol and drug addiction,
and for those who treat them*

Contents

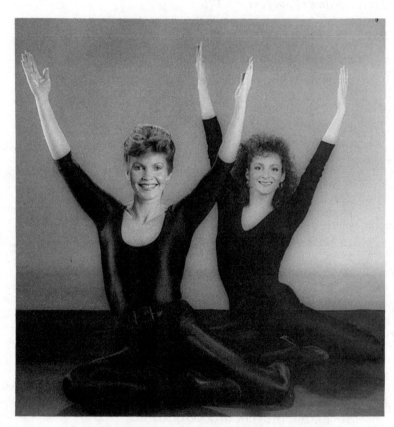

Judy Myers and her daughter Julietta Marcelli

Foreword

Staying Sober is not just another dissertation on the evils and pitfalls of alcoholism and drug addiction. Judy Myers has captured the essential secrets of recovery by combining pure science, the precepts of Alcoholics Anonymous, and specific nutrition and fitness activities that will ensure recovery. Her Recovery/Relapse-Prevention Program is the first blueprint to achieving recovery and maintaining it for a lifetime. Thrown in for good measure are tips on how to achieve a terrific appearance, good stamina, and a positive attitude. Judy Myers has managed to capture the practical essence of what the research scientists have been saying in recent years as to what is necessary to maintain recovery.

The person who becomes an alcoholic or drug addict may be born with certain genetic defects of the neurochemical system. Once the abuse of alcohol or drugs is chronic, the neurochemical defects become more aggravated. According to a growing body of scientific research, those defects may become permanent.

Judy Myers doesn't·hide behind a curtain of denial. She comes right out and says that the only real way to control the neurochemical changes that alcoholism and addiction produce is through specific nutritional habits, health behaviors, and exercise. She eloquently states that Alcoholics Anonymous is a valuable first step, but lifelong recovery will likely require a thorough program of nutrition and exercise. She labels this the "missing link." Nothing could be more correct. The nutritional guidelines and exercise program described in this book will help recovering individuals maximize their brain and neurochemical systems not only to maintain recovery but to maintain it in a way that permits happiness and a fulfilling life.

This book is "must" reading for anyone who is in a recovery program or for anyone who has a friend or loved one who wants to recover. I also recommend this book to any professional who wants to help people achieve and maintain recovery, since it contains many helpful ideas.

FOREST TENNANT, M.D., D.P.H.
EXECUTIVE DIRECTOR, COMMUNITY HEALTH PROJECTS
DRUG ADVISOR FOR THE NATIONAL FOOTBALL LEAGUE
AND THE LOS ANGELES DODGERS

Acknowledgments

I want to give a special thanks to my family, especially my children, Michael and Julietta, who have provided me with the support and encouragement to complete this task. I thank Alcoholics Anonymous for saving my life. Thanks to Jim Wilkerson, Medrick Rue, Carl Chandler, Evie Romero, Jackie Gershen, Dawn House, Tim Schreiber, Catherine Paura, "Christmas Tree Helen," "Boston Helen," Don Bauder, all the people at the Beverly Hills Sports Connection, Dr. Howard Hunt, Elaine Lane, Rick Dees, Dr. Sheldon Hendler, Dr. Forest Tennant, Dr. Eula West, John Gates, Rafer Johnson, Gil Clancy, Cory Everson, Ellen Kelleher, Bob Earl, Pastor Jack Hayford of Church on the Way, Pastor Jerry Barnard of Christian Communications Network, and all my clients.

Thanks to my co-writer, Maribeth Mellin, who made the book "sing." I also want to extend a special thank-you to my agent, Mark McCormack, president and CEO of International Management Group, who believed in me and this project. Included in this assistance were Angela Miller, Dave Gibbons, Bev Norwood, and Erik Van Dillen.

Most of all, I am grateful to my Higher Power, whom I call God, who gave me the wisdom, inspiration, and guidance to produce this book.

JUDY MYERS

Judy Myers created this concept and book; I thank her for trusting me to understand its importance. Richard Louv taught me to be a writer. Jane Onstott provided encouragement, support, and assistance with the last-minute details; Dan Janeck gave editorial guidance and many hours at the computer. Most of all, I thank the people in my own life who have struggled with and overcome the disease and far-reaching fallout of alcoholism. Their example has taught me much about courage, wisdom, and self-respect.

MARIBETH MELLIN

CREDITS:

AVIA Footwear
Gold's Gym, Venice, California
Lance Gavin Strugar, hairstylist
Leigh Charlton, makeup artist

Who hath woe? Who hath sorrow?

Who hath contentions?
Who hath babbling?
Who hath wounds without cause?
Who hath redness of the eyes?
They that tarry long at the wine.
At last it biteth like a serpent
And stingeth like an adder.
Thine eyes shall behold strange women,
And thy heart shall utter perverse things.
They have stricken me, shalt thou say
And I was not sick;
They have beaten me,
And I felt it not;
When shall I wake?

I will seek it yet again.

PROVERBS 23:29

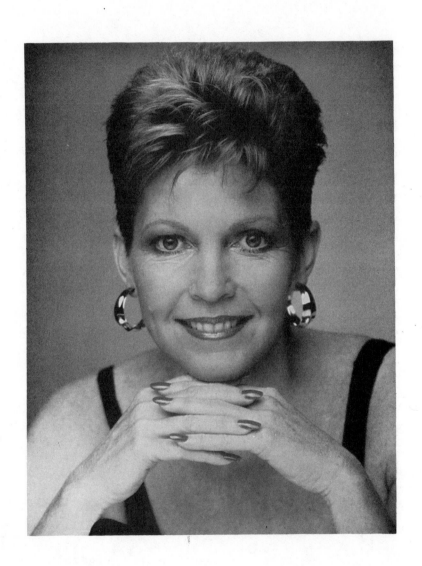

Introduction

*I*am a recovering alcoholic. I have been drunk, broken, desperate, and alone. I have been treated by psychologists, psychiatrists, physicians, and ministers. I have been hospitalized, institutionalized, detoxified, ostracized. I have been hung over, dried out, sober, and drunk all in the same day, over and over again. I have recovered, relapsed, and recovered so often the cycle became the norm. My life was a series of deliriums.

Why couldn't I stop? Why did I repeatedly return to self-destruction, embracing my desperation? Why did misery seem stronger than hope?

THE LIMITS OF DETOXIFICATION

It happened because my healers assumed detoxification would be my salvation. They ignored the reality that life remains the same long after the tremors have stopped. They forgot the causes and effects of my addiction. They eliminated the poison but gave me nothing to take its place. They took away my constant companion and left me alone.

1

I was no longer addicted, but I was still imprisoned by defeat. I had forgotten how it felt to be healthy, happy, and truly alive.

I entered a recovery house in San Diego, determined to remember what I had lost. I was told that one key to successful sobriety was working with other alcoholics. I agreed, but wondered what I could possibly offer them. I reviewed the house's program and finally discovered the missing link. No one had thought to teach recovering alcoholics how to repair their bodies and prepare their minds for future challenges and defeats.

They had ignored a most critical element of success—optimal physical condition and healthful nutrition. As a former health and physical education teacher, I knew the importance of diet and exercise. Yet even I had overlooked the absolute necessity of rebuilding my body and recapturing the multiple benefits of health.

Current detoxification programs do "dry out" their patients; in that sense, they meet their goal. But sober alcoholics remain marooned in unhealthy, destructive lifestyles. They still have terrible eating habits, made worse by substitute addictions to caffeine, nicotine, and sugar. Their harmful habits make sleep irregular at best, causing their health to deteriorate even further.

Having escaped from a drug- and alcohol-dependent world, they are suddenly set adrift in a dry world without direction, discipline, or purpose. Their ability to cope with stress and emotional upheaval is negligible: no one teaches them how to replace the anesthetics they have been using to dull the daily traumas of life. They hang on to sobriety with uncertainty, full of fear and doubt, hoping to be rescued from their anxieties before they succumb to the familiar comforts of alcohol and drugs.

THE PATH TO RECOVERY

This realization became the fuel for my recovery and the inspiration for my future success. I worked with the other women at the house, teaching them how to exercise, eat right, and gain a positive outlook on life. I left there healthier and happier than I had felt in years, with a new sense of purpose and possibility. I began working with other recovering alcoholics and addicts, individually and in hospitals and treatment centers. Every one of these people needed exercise, proper nutrition, motivation, and guidance for a new and healthy life. I provided tailor-made regimes based on each person's physical, mental, and emotional condition. I watched people who had repeatedly relapsed into addiction gain a sense of self-confidence and self-respect that allowed them to remain healthy and free.

The path from addiction to recovery is not a natural one. It is fraught with dangerous traps and debilitating drawbacks. It is the loneliest, most frightening road a person can take. At the beginning, the dependence on alcohol and drugs seems so much easier and more comforting than independence and health. But death is addiction's only reward.

Alcoholics Anonymous, Narcotics Anonymous, and their off-shoots give alcoholics and addicts spiritual direction, companionship, encouragement, and a blueprint for life. It is quite possible that A.A. has saved your life. I know it saved mine. I believe in the power of A.A. Its traditions, steps, and members are the foundation of my life in recovery.

As an adjunct to programs such as A.A., the Recovery/Relapse-Prevention Program described in this book empowers alcoholics and addicts. It gives them responsibility for their recovery with clear, concise, competent directions for success. It teaches them to appreciate their strengths, amplify their abilities, and allow themselves the blessings of self-respect. It gives them the one thing they need most—the missing link to recovery for life.

Alcoholics and addicts can regain self-control and pride. The process requires basic fitness and nutrition tenets that are generally not available. This program can save lives and forever end the cycle of wet and dry, clean and dirty, straight and relapsed. There is a way. That's why I wrote this book.

THE NEED

It is impossible to adequately calculate the number of alcoholics and drug addicts in this country or in the world. It is safe to assume that the numbers are enormous and increase daily. Alcoholism and drug addiction are newsworthy; barely a week goes by without concentrated media attention on some aspect of these diseases, which threaten all our lives.

Major athletic organizations have finally become cognizant of the scores of addicts in their ranks, through the death of basketball star Len Bias and the destruction of other promising young athletes. Military institutions regularly screen their personnel for drug and alcohol use; corporations have instituted recovery programs; insurance companies are becoming more willing to provide coverage for treatment of alcoholism and drug addiction. The president has called for a "War on Drugs." Suspicion and paranoia have invaded our right to privacy and our sense of community.

As the furor against alcohol and drugs mounts, alcoholics and addicts have become more willing to publicly acknowledge their afflictions. Gradually, we as a society are realizing that punishment is not a cure, that addiction is not an issue of us against them. We are all harmed by these diseases. Yet much of what is done for those who are addicted concentrates solely on eliminating the addiction rather than healing the addict.

The Recovery/Relapse-Prevention Program takes up where most of the existing recovery programs for addicts fall short. It combines the physical, mental, and spiritual elements of our disease and recovery. To have total, long-lasting recovery, all three aspects must be addressed. You can't expect success if you fix one and ignore the others.

Fitness, nutrition, and stress management are critical to the treatment of any disease. They are imperative when dealing with a disease that necessitates intensive changes in lifestyle. No one can or will give up an addiction that provides temporary relief unless he or she can replace it with permanent health and well-being. My program gives recovering alcoholics and addicts the information and guidance they need to rebuild their bodies and minds and to reshape their lifestyles in a happy, healthy manner.

A GUIDE FOR YOU

This book was written for you. Though all of us as alcoholics and addicts suffer from the same disease, we are each unique. We have our own highly personal problems, sorrows, values, and strengths. We will not all recover in the same way. But we can use the same tools.

The Recovery/Relapse-Prevention (RRP) Program is your guide to a healthy recovery. With it, you can design a personalized fitness and nutrition program that suits your body, personality, and lifestyle. I recommend that you read this book from start to finish, without doing the assignments or filling out the worksheets. Then start your Recovery/Relapse-Prevention notebook, using whatever format works best for you. Read each chapter again, closely, and complete the assignments and worksheets in Appendix A (pages 181–240). Give yourself plenty of time for this process of self-evaluation. When you finish, you will have organized your RRP Program and will be ready to implement it.

Stick with your program for thirty days, then retest yourself. You will see dramatic changes and know you are well on your way toward fitness and health.

As you follow your RRP Program, you will eliminate the notion that achieving health has to be painful. Use the hints this book offers to find out what works best for you. Listen to your body. You will learn that it is possible to feel wonderful and take care of yourself simultaneously. You won't have to "go for the burn" or eat flavorless foods to get healthy and fit. You will have fun as you take charge of your recovery and regain your health.

Those who cannot enter treatment programs because they lack money, insurance, or available programs can, with the help of their doctor, implement the Recovery/Relapse-Prevention Program as an alternative. In that situation, the backup support of A.A. or a similar group is especially important.

I am a recovering alcoholic who has spent most of her adult life as a health and physical education teacher. My program, which evolved through my recovery, teaches you a step-by-step, day-by-day method for achieving and maintaining fitness and health. You can recover and experience optimal health. I've done it, my clients have done it, and so will you.

PART I

NUTRITION

We drank for joy and became miserable.
We drank for sociability and became argumentative.
We drank for sophistication and became obnoxious.
We drank for friendship and became enemies.
We drank to help us sleep and awakened exhausted.
We drank to gain strength and it made us weaker.
We drank for exhilaration and ended up depressed.
We drank for "medical reasons" and acquired health
    problems.
We drank to help us calm down and ended up with the
    shakes.
We drank to get more confidence and became afraid.
We drank to make conversation flow more easily and the
    words came out slurred and incoherent.
We drank to diminish our problems and saw them
    multiply.
We drank to feel heavenly and ended up feeling like hell.

AUTHOR UNKNOWN

1
King Alcohol

*M*y first day at the recovery house still burns in my memory. I had hit bottom. I was physically, mentally, and spiritually bankrupt. I was an alcoholic. I had finally conceded that my life was out of control.

What a change that was for the athlete who loved to compete and win. Could I come out on top this time? As I quickly learned in A.A., the opponent was a monster—cunning, powerful, baffling, and totally destructive. King Alcohol. I decided to go to any lengths to beat this deadly opponent. My sponsor at A.A. suggested I move into a recovery home, where the weapons for my war would be provided. Little did I know the impact these battles would have on my life and the lives of others.

When I arrived, I faced six women sitting in a circle, waiting for their A.A. meeting to start. As we surveyed each other, I wondered about their pasts. Had they suffered as much as I? I doubted it.

I had been a winner. Wealthy, attractive, successful in business and relationships. I lived in a $500,000 penthouse overlooking the Pacific Ocean and worked at a lucrative business I had created by myself.

9

FROM SUCCESS TO DESTITUTION

It took years of hard work to build my company, and only hours to destroy it. I had taken on a partner—a charming, capable con man who absconded with everything I owned, including my clothes. I went from riches to destitution in one short day. Within a month I was forced to move to a small studio apartment. I was broke and broken, so devastated that I drank to ease the pain. At first I drank socially, commiserating with companions at parties and bars. Then I drank at home, alone, all day and all night. The blackouts began, with their unforgiving hangovers, fatigue, anxiety, and unrelenting guilt. Everything I touched turned to dust. The super saleswoman of yesterday couldn't sell a life preserver to a drowning man.

I visited a psychiatrist, who asked me if I drank. "Of course not," I replied. He said I was suffering from severe depression and sent me to a hospital for four weeks. There I met a patient from the alcoholic ward. I taught him how to play tennis and took him to my church. He invited me to an A.A. meeting. I told him I didn't drink, but would join him out of curiosity. Lies came easily then. I went to the meeting, and left with the nagging realization that I was probably an alcoholic. I kept that knowledge to myself. A few weeks later, after my release from the hospital, I noticed some A.A. pamphlets in my psychiatrist's waiting room. I stuck some in my purse—just out of curiosity.

The pamphlets listed the locations and times of A.A. meetings in San Diego, including one right across the street from where I lived. I knew I had a choice—go meet my friends at the neighborhood hangout or go to the meeting across the street. I don't know what came over me. I don't know where I got the strength. But I grabbed my purse and ran across the street to my first A.A. meeting as an honest alcoholic. Just a few weeks later, I was facing the women who would become my housemates, my students, and my friends during the most painful transformation of my life.

"WHAT WAS IT LIKE?"

The recovery house director brought me back to reality as she
began the A.A. meeting by asking each of us, "What was it like
before you came here? How do you feel now?"

Sue was 28 and very overweight. She had short, dirty blond hair
and was wearing wrinkled chinos and a stained white sweatshirt.
Her career as the agent for a famous European rock singer had
crashed after she was introduced to cocaine and alcohol. After five
years, the drugs and chaotic lifestyle had worn her down. She was
fired from her job. Her family considered her an embarrassment
and banished her from their home. She no longer had the money to
support her addictions.

She discovered A.A. in France and collected enough money to
move to California to dry out. The hospital she ended up in
transferred her to this home, where she talked about how grateful
she was to be drug-free and sober. Now she wanted to lose weight
and gain energy. She had gained 40 pounds in five months because
of her uncontrollable urge for chocolate. We didn't understand it at
the time, but sugar had become her substitute addiction, still
robbing her of happiness and health.

Annie, who was only 20 years old, told her story next. Four
months before, she had been arrested for public drunkenness and
placed in a detoxification center, then transferred to the recovery
house. Three years earlier, during the Christmas holidays, Annie's
parents were killed in a head-on traffic collision. The people she
met in bars became her new family. But now she said she had
found her real family in A.A. She talked about her violent mood
swings and long periods of depression. She thought she was
overweight, and wanted to quit smoking and stop eating sugar.
Could her emotional problems have been the by-products of an
alcoholic's typically poor nutrition?

A beautiful blonde woman in her early 30s spoke next. She had
owned a successful salon at the beach but lost it when she
squandered her profits on cocaine and expensive liquor. She was

back at the recovery house for her second time, saying she hoped it would be her last. Her real name was Lillian, but she preferred to be called Lynn. Her hands shook as she tried to light a cigarette. She choked as she spoke of the shame of spending a night in detox. All she wanted, she said, was to get sober, lose weight, and feel good about herself again.

Maria, who was in her late 20s, raised her hand to speak next. She started crying as she showed us pictures of her children. They were living in foster homes; she was not allowed to see them. She lived on alcohol and downers and had come to the home from a psychiatric hospital where she had been placed after attempting suicide. Maria was at least 20 pounds overweight and constantly depressed. She hated being in the recovery house but had stayed sober for two and a half months.

A woman who appeared to be in her late 60s sat apart from the group in a corner. She couldn't have weighed more than 80 pounds, and looked terribly frightened and fragile. At first she declined to speak but finally responded to the director's prodding. In a voice barely louder than a whisper, Alice told us she had been sober for 16 years. Then she started working overtime as an excuse to miss her A.A. meetings. Before long, her obsession for alcohol returned. One drink led to another, and she could no longer stay sober. She lectured the rest of us on the dangers of stress, and pointed out the wisdom of the A.A. slogan "easy does it." She was a widow, lived alone, and had stopped eating regularly. I wondered if she was healthy enough to make it through the program. She said she was fearful but grateful to be with us.

The last woman to speak was a feisty redhead who had encouraged the others to speak out. Jill was in her early 40s and said she was going through a divorce and was back in recovery for the second time. She had been there seven months.

THE FAILURE FACTOR

I wondered why she had returned and stayed for so long. Seven months? As I looked at the other repeaters I kept wondering,

"Why?" Slowly, the failure factor began to sink in. So many relapses, so many returns. What was missing? I asked Jill.

She said she had had a good job as a loan officer at a bank. She went to work drunk and was fired. Her husband locked her out of the house, yelling, "I don't want a fat, drunk broad for a wife!" Their 10-year marriage was over, and she was devastated. She said she hoped to get her husband back by staying sober, losing weight, and getting a good job at another bank. She had been at the home long enough to become the resident manager. She said she was happy to be sober, but wanted to leave the home as soon as possible and never return.

Every woman there had a different story. All had suffered immense losses; all shared the same basic hope. We wanted to feel better, look better, and remain sober. I knew we could all be in better physical shape.

I looked back on the depressions that were brought on by drinking. I had had severe headaches and always had seemed to have had some kind of flu or bronchitis. My face was puffy; my body looked bloated. I was surprised to learn that the other women looked and felt the same. Even though we were all sober, we were neither healthy nor happy. What was missing?

FINDING THE MISSING LINK

Our common malaise reawakened my interest in fitness and nutrition. I remembered how I tried to stay slim by not eating because I knew there were a lot of calories in alcohol. I semistarved myself, then binged on junk food. I resolved to use my time in recovery to get my body back in shape and start eating right again. Even at that early stage, I knew intuitively that poor nutrition was a major obstacle to recovery. I wanted to become an expert.

I began monitoring my behavior closely. I noticed how I instinctively reached for chocolates, how I lusted for french fries, doughnuts, and greasy foods. I felt proud when I refused to succumb to those temptations. I recognized sugar as an enemy.

The more I studied nutrition, the more I learned about sugar's insidious role in alcoholism. I learned that most recovering alcoholics suffer from low blood sugar and try to gain quick energy from candy bars and cookies. I formulated a diet that counteracted this tendency and slowly developed my own eating plan. I understood my depression and how it was caused by the internal damages of alcohol.

The other stumbling block to recovery was my poor physical condition. I remembered how good I felt when I was in shape. Through research I learned that medical experts were discovering that fitness was indeed a key to recovery. In fact, fitness was not merely a key. It was the missing link.

I decided to jog around the block every morning. The first time I tried, I could only go halfway. I couldn't believe how out of shape I'd become. It took two weeks before I could make it around without struggling. But once I did it, I felt a tremendous sense of achievement. There was a beautiful park nearby with a one-and-a-half-mile trail. During my third week of running, I tried out the trail—one-third running, one-third walking, one-third running. It was wonderful!

I could see and almost feel the control I had gained over my life once again. As my physical condition improved, my bouts of depression diminished. The zest I felt after each workout pulsed in my veins as if life itself had been transfused into me. Was that physiologically possible? Yes. Research now indicates that exercise is as vital to recovering alcoholics as food is to the starving. The benefits I felt were not only the general results of physical fitness. There were important chemical and physiological changes taking place in my body—changes that only exercise could provide. Only exercise could reverse the damage caused by my disease—the disease of addiction.

My outlook turned from despair to euphoria in only one month. The other women were still wrestling with depression and inertia. My fitness program was the only thing that separated me from them.

After five weeks, I had lost eight pounds. My enthusiasm was becoming contagious, and my friends were pleading for my help. They all wanted what I had attained. They wanted more than the weight loss and physical conditioning. They envied the control I was exerting over my existence.

At first I was reluctant to assume the role of their fitness guru. I still wasn't all that used to controlling my own life. But as I took them under my newfound wing of health, I realized the reason I was there. I finally had a purpose and a strong sense of hope.

FITNESS TEAMWORK

Our first session started in the park. We couldn't just take off and run—their muscles were frozen from lack of use. I began with a few warm-up exercises and smiled at the moans as they stretched. Some of those rebellious muscles resented their reawakening. I taught the women to start slowly, to pace themselves, and to appreciate every moment of progress.

As the weeks went by, their enthusiasm grew. We rejoiced together, feeling much better than we had in years. They told me their depressions were lifting and their flab was disappearing. Those parasitic demons of fear and anxiety also were being exorcised by exercise. I beamed with the satisfaction that only comes to a human who helps other humans.

A leaflet announcing the Alcoholic Olympics arrived at the home. I told the women about this annual event and how it was designed to honor recovering alcoholics and addicts. They reacted with fear and refused to participate. I realized I had some selling to do. I told them the importance lay in the trying, not the winning. I explained that it was vitally important for them to transfer their rediscovered energy into other aspects of their lives. I said it was time to take a step outside the cozy confines of our protected environment. Eventually, we were all going to have to take risks in order to survive. This was a way to start, I said, but we had to commit ourselves soon. The Olympics were only four weeks away. They said they would think about it.

The following week I used our running time to continue my lecture, trying to convince them that the Olympics were important. They did not respond. I knew I had to be silent while the challenge percolated in their minds. Two weeks later, as we met for our morning run, they announced that they were willing to participate. "All right!" I shouted in delight, leading our team down the familiar path.

That night we discussed the events. I described the fun run, the long jump, and the relay race. We chose our events and geared ourselves up for competition.

Although we came from divergent backgrounds, we had grown as close as sisters in our group battle against addiction. We learned the value of teamwork and a sense of community, both of which had been missing in our lives. The common lot of drinkers is isolation and a terrible loneliness. We were discarding that lifestyle with our interest in physical conditioning and nutrition and our present involvement in a community event, the Alcoholic Olympics.

THE ALCOHOLIC OLYMPICS

I will never forget that day. Almost 6,000 recovering alcoholics, drug addicts, and supporters were there, representing 20 rehabilitation and treatment centers. Each team carried its banner as we marched around the college stadium to the cadence of the Marine Corps band. The Olympics' motto hung over the stadium: "To Try Is to Win." We were convinced.

We all entered the first event, a three-and-a-half-mile fun run. Halfway throught the race, I ran out of energy and did a slow jog to the finish line. When I reached the end, one of the last across the line, the other women were cheering me on, ignoring the fact that they'd beaten their coach. As I wiped the sweat from my eyes, I realized Sue was cradling a huge trophy in her arms. She was screaming with joy, jumping up and down, tears streaming down her cheeks.

"I won! I won! I've never won anything in my whole life! And I did it just for me!"

I looked at the other women and realized each had won a medal for her age group. They were delirious with excitement and accomplishment. Yes, Sue had won for herself. She had won back her self-esteem, lost her unwanted pounds, and gained the benefits of good nutrition and health. The other women shared her joy and pride.

By the end of the day, I had won four gold medals, and each of the other women had won three. Our small group had racked up enough team points to win second place.

The games underscored my belief in the importance of fitness and nutrition for the recovering alcoholic and drug addict. My decision to make this my life's work was now irrevocable. I dove into my future with a missionary's zeal.

After I left the recovery home, I volunteered in hospitals and detoxification centers. These places provided little in the way of fitness programs, and nutritional education was either absent or obsolete. I realized that precious little was being done to help addicts change their lifestyles. Many of the people who became detoxified soon succumbed to other diseases caused by poor nutrition, smoking, or other forms of self-abuse. The percentage of relapses was staggering. In contrast, the women from the home, including myself, had all remained sober, straight, and successful.

Alcoholics and addicts can live healthy, happy lives. They can combine spiritual, mental, and physical healing and take charge of their souls, minds, and bodies. My RRP Program can help show the way.

2
The Addicted Body

I believe I was born an alcoholic." Every alcoholic has made that statement at some time, and with good reason. Ongoing research confirms the physiological causes and effects of addiction. The scientific evidence repeatedly bolsters our belief that we have a physical disease, not a psychological weakness. Our gut-level fears and instincts just might be correct.

ALCOHOLISM AND GENETICS

If alcoholism is a physiological disorder, are we born with a predisposition to addiction? Can alcoholism be inherited? Recent studies by psychiatrist Donald Goodwin, whose results are included in his book *Is Alcoholism Hereditary?*, provide clear and strong corroboration that alcoholism is passed from parent to child through the genes.

Like many alcoholics, I need only look at my family to reinforce my belief in the reality of the genetic transference of alcoholism; the disease indeed seems to be passed from generation to generation.

18

While I was living in the recovery house, rebuilding my life, I asked my mother to tell my twin brother, Dennis, and my older brother, Peter, that I was an alcoholic. A few weeks later, Dennis called and told me he had recently joined A.A. in San Jose. Though our lives and lifestyles were radically different, though we rarely saw or spoke with each other, we were living the same nightmare. Peter called a few days later and told me he had joined Overeaters Anonymous and was "visiting" A.A.

I started wondering about my father. We had stopped living together when I was eight years old; in the past few years, I had completely lost contact with him. After I left the recovery house and felt I was in control of my life, I visited my father in San Francisco. One evening, when we were alone, he asked if it was true that I was in A.A. I was embarrassed and scared as I hesitantly said, "Yes. Yes I am." He looked at me and smiled in recognition and delight. With a little boy's glee in his voice and a familiar Irish sparkle in his eyes he yelled, "So am I!"

As Goodwin says in his book, "The 'Father's sins' may be visited on the sons even in the father's absence." We discovered, in a rush of confidences, that he had joined A.A. 60 days after I had. Dennis had joined 30 days after him; Peter started visiting meetings at the same time. In three months the four of us, living in four different cities, oblivious to each others' lives, had faced our alcoholism and decided to conquer it. As far as I was concerned, the evidence was overwhelming. We were a family bonded by blood and alcohol.

My father, my brothers, and I had nearly simultaneously achieved the first step of A.A.: "We admitted we were powerless over alcohol—that our lives had become unmanageable." It may have taken many years of illness, heartbreak, and destruction to reach that initial step toward happiness and health, but we did it, apart and together.

AN ONSLAUGHT OF ABUSE

Our bodies (and souls and spirits and minds) endure a tremendous onslaught of abuse as we alcoholics avoid the realities of our disease. I realized the full impact of that abuse while working with the women at the recovery home. No matter what type of recovery program they had attended, no matter how long they had been sober, they were still in miserable physical shape, still far from healthy.

"I am an alcoholic and a drug addict." That phrase echoes through A.A. meetings wherever I go, like a universal chant. Often, those of us who are addicted to alcohol say we started using drugs when our drinking interfered with our social and professional lives. We went to doctors and described our symptoms—nervousness, anxiety, insomnia, fatigue, mysterious aches and pains, weight losses and gains—and got tranquilizers, sedatives, barbiturates, sleeping pills, pain pills, diet pills, antidepressants, mood elevators. We faithfully took all our medications as prescribed, adding to our pill stash every time we visited a new physician. Or we turned to the street, to our drinking buddies, for cocaine, marijuana, speed, uppers, downers—any drug that could mask our discomfort. Anything to nourish the deadly false image of pleasure.

"Anything in excess of two, I am addicted to." Some of us used drugs to get off alcohol; others used alcohol to get off drugs. Neither technique proved successful. They only amplified our disease into multiple addictions, further destroying our bodies, making our withdrawal even more difficult and painful. If we wanted to be sober and clean, we faced the possibility of enduring increased anxiety, tremors, weakness, nausea, vomiting, sweating, convulsions, delirium tremens (DTs), confusion, disorientation, and hallucinations. Is it any wonder that in order to recover fully, we must get our bodies, minds, and spirits fit?

THE BODY'S RESPONSES

The insidious, long-term effects of alcoholism start eating away at our well-being long, long before we notice our health deteriorating.

Drug addiction magnifies and accelerates the damage, adding deadly items to our lists of wounds. The list is long enough with alcohol alone.

Our bodies adjust cooperatively to alcohol, and demand more in order to operate efficiently. Our cells use alcohol as an energy source; our tolerance increases. Often, it is not until we stop drinking that we realize how much our bodies depend on alcohol. Then, when the nausea, sweats, tremors, and paranoia hit, we have proof that we feel better when we drink, proof that we need alcohol. Proof that without alcohol, we need drugs.

We do not automatically heal when we stop drinking. The alcohol and other drugs we have consumed have wreaked havoc throughout our bodies. The effects stay with us long after we recognize and deal with our disease. The first year is the hardest. Though we are eager to begin changing our lives, the alcohol and its effects are still in our bodies, altering our decision-making abilities. Fortunately, just as we have learned to stop drinking, we can learn to regain our health. Proper nutrition and adequate exercise, geared to the needs of the recovering alcoholic, can significantly lessen our bodies' dependence on alcohol and prevent further dependence on drugs, caffeine, and sugar.

First, we must recognize the ways in which alcohol has damaged our bodies. The physical and psychological effects of alcoholism are numerous. Many of the most common ones are described in the following paragraphs.

Psychological Problems. Psychological problems associated with alcoholism include anxiety, depression, blackouts, personality disorders, and all the psychological symptoms that cause so many of us to think we suffer from a mental disease and say we should be able to will away our thirst for alcohol. Alcohol (ethanol) is a general anesthetic. It depresses the central nervous system and inhibits proper brain functioning. At its most toxic levels, it can cause permanent brain damage. It robs the brain of essential nutrients, causing alcoholics to act bizarre and irrational.

Malnutrition, Digestive Problems, and Eating Disorders. In *Dr. Atkins' Nutrition Breakthrough*, Dr. Robert Atkins calls alcohol an "antinutrient." We suffer from malnutrition because our bodies have lost the ability to absorb, utilize, and store nutrients, which are responsible for the growth, maintenance, and repair of our damaged tissues and organs. Alcohol masks the signals of hunger and appetite. The central nervous system and the liver adapt so well to abuse that they keep us dependent on alcohol, further degrading our nutritional well-being.

Since alcohol contains calories, it may be referred to as a food and can be used by the body to produce energy. When we receive a major portion of our caloric intake from alcohol, our demands for food diminish. Some alcoholics lose their appetites completely, even after they are sober. Twenty ounces of 86-proof whiskey contain approximately 1,500 calories—all the calories a grown woman needs to survive. Those of us who are vain about our weight think that if we consume large amounts of alcohol, there is little need to eat. This is about as effective as changing deck chairs on the *Titanic*. We are consuming empty calories—no proteins, vitamins, or nutrients—using a poison that easily destroys our fragile health. We are as malnourished as starving children.

Prolonged use of alcohol causes irritation and inflammation of the stomach lining causing gastritis and other digestive problems.

Liver Dysfunction, Hepatitis, Cirrhosis. Research suggests that alcoholics have a liver cell malfunction; from the time we start drinking, our liver cells adapt to alcohol and continue adapting, increasing our tolerance for alcohol. We drink more, and the liver works harder, destroying itself. The liver is essential for the storage and metabolism of nutrients. As it concentrates on metabolizing alcohol, which distorts and kills its cells, the liver becomes less efficient at metabolizing healthful nutrients. It is possible for the liver to build new cells and fight damage, but only if it is fed the proper nutrients and allowed to return to some semblance of normal functioning.

Disorders of the Heart and Circulatory System. Alcoholics are susceptible to high blood pressure, cardiac irregularities, heart attacks, strokes, and anemia. Mineral, vitamin, and protein deficiencies weaken the heart muscles and prohibit the proper synthesis of proteins, leading to impaired cardiac functioning. Since alcohol inhibits the liver's ability to metabolize fats, cholesterol and triglyceride levels in the blood increase, thus clogging and eventually hardening the arteries. Red blood cells become distorted and die when iron and other minerals are not properly metabolized, and the alcoholic becomes anemic, fatigued, and sedentary, further limiting the heart's efficiency.

Hypoglycemia. Alcoholics trying to stay sober often become sugar addicts—we crave sugar the way we once craved alcohol, and become frustrated when we can't will ourselves away from chocolate and sweets. We get tired, shaky, depressed, anxious, and hungry, and we know sugar will jolt those symptoms away, temporarily. We are suffering, once again, from a metabolic disorder—chronic low blood sugar, or hypoglycemia. "An alcoholic who switches his addiction to sweets can be just as moody, unstable and exhausted as when he was drinking," Dr. Atkins writes. "If the former alcoholic stays addicted to sugar, I believe there is a greater chance of his returning to the bottle than if he kicks both alcohol and sweets and keeps his blood sugar stable."

Our bodies are equipped to handle an occasional strain in the form of excess sugar. The pancreas produces insulin, which is released into the bloodstream, where it destroys the excess sugar. But if we continuously bombard our systems with large amounts of easily absorbed sugar, our sugar-regulating mechanisms become damaged and even destroyed. When insulin is released into the bloodstream to counteract the high sugar level, it quickly drops the sugar level far below normal. Heart and muscle performance weakens. Brain and nerve performance is damaged. Energy and endurance levels fall drastically. Emotional stability and control disappear. We crave a quick pickup from sweets, coffee, alcohol, or certain drugs that rapidly remedy the unpleasant symptoms by bringing up the blood sugar level. The pancreas is once again called upon to overreact and counteract the new onslaught of sugar; it again overproduces insulin.

We are victims of this vicious cycle—hyperactive, happy, and energetic for a short time when the sugar level is high; and totally exhausted, confused, and ready to leap out of our skin a few hours later. Eating sugar or taking a drink will not help the situation. Eating the proper amounts of protein, carbohydrates, and natural sugars will help immensely, and specific nutritional supplements can help curb sugar cravings.

Aches and Injuries. Alcoholics are also susceptible to frequent head and body aches, fractures, sprains, and serious injuries. The state of drunkenness leads to increased physical damage from easily avoided accidents. Again, the inability of the body to properly metabolize nutrients causes the muscles and bones to weaken and become susceptible to injury.

Other Symptoms. Frequent colds, respiratory infections, digestive disorders, nightmares, insomnia, blackouts, bloatedness, skin rashes, blotches, broken blood vessels, wrinkles and lines—the list is endless. The ravages are self-evident. We who have suffered alcohol and chemical torture and are willing to go to any lengths to stay sober can understand how alcohol has damaged us and learn how to heal and prevent further damage from relapses. We can repair our diseased bodies and live our lives to their fullest. And, in the tradition of successful sobriety, we can help each other toward health, happiness, and well-being.

THE BENEFITS OF FITNESS

The benefits of exercise and proper nutrition are easy to see. Your liver cleans itself, and your heart becomes a strong and powerful muscle, pumping efficiently. Your lungs turn pink, fed by vitamins and fresh air. Your brain works with the clarity of freedom and health, no longer befuddled by battling chemicals. You sleep at night, all night, free of nightmares, sweats, and sudden cravings. Your hair shines, your skin glows, you move with a sense of worth.

You have learned a life-giving lesson. You have finally realized that you are not a bad person trying to be good. You are a sick person trying to get well. And you are succeeding.

ASSIGNMENTS

1. Begin your RRP Program notebook. I find that a spiral notebook works best for me, but you may prefer a looseleaf notebook, or even a computer file. Whatever you choose, it should be compact enough for you to keep with you at all times. You will use this notebook to record your answers to the worksheets and self-evaluations, to plan your nutrition and fitness programs, and to record your observations, goals, and successes.

2. Take a picture of yourself, facing the camera, head to toe. Hang it somewhere where you will see it often, or mount it in your Recovery/Relapse-Prevention Program notebook.

3
Your Nutritional Guidelines

*I*magine waking up cheerful in the morning, humming in the shower, smiling at the mirror, knowing your good humor will last through the day. Your clothes slide easily over your limber frame. You walk with confidence.

Snap this picture in your memory. Find a saying, a scene, a person who reminds you of yourself at your best. Hang it near the self-portrait you made as you finished reading Chapter 2. Start loading your mind, home, and workplace with positive signals— whatever works best for you. Decide that you can gradually transform your self-portrait into the picture in your imagination.

EASING INTO SOBRIETY

The Recovery/Relapse-Prevention Program is not a diet. It is a lifestyle, to be adopted gradually. You may have kicked alcohol or drugs cold turkey, and do best when you set absolute goals. If so, clean out your refrigerator and cabinets and wave good-bye to your food addictions. You may instead be terrified at the thought of never eating sugar—no brownies, ice cream, or candy. Easy does it. You're probably a one-day-at-a-time person. Take the time to learn what works best for you.

You now know, from reading about your addicted body, that your tissues, organs, muscles, bones, and brain have taken a beating from alcohol. You may not know what health feels like. I assure you, it feels great. I look at myself, my clients, and my recovering friends and see striking changes in our moods, attitudes, and self-respect. I know health is possible; I know it is wonderful.

And I know it takes time, and no small measure of frustration, to build and maintain a healthy body. The RRP Program is designed to help you ease into a healthy sobriety and minimize the cravings that make relapses so dangerous.

This plan for health and sobriety is threefold. The first step is recognizing and halting your addiction. People in A.A. have most likely learned to believe in and seek the help of a Higher Power and other recovering alcoholics. They know that A.A. is a part of their life, forever. Here you will learn about the two other steps that you can incorporate into your lives to help you recover and stay sober, healthy, and happy—nutrition and fitness.

HOW NUTRITION CAN REMEDY ALCOHOL AND CHEMICAL ABUSE

It is not easy to change lifelong eating patterns, but it is worthwhile. Your life can be transformed. You will feel better, maybe better than ever, and you will probably save thousands of dollars on medical bills. Chances are good you will live longer, and be happy about that. You will gain health, prevent relapse, and ward off illness. You will decrease your depressions, increase your stamina, and look better and younger.

Nutrition will not turn back any clocks. Some of the physical wounds from alcohol cannot be eliminated. If you are suffering from cirrhosis, hepatitis, gastritis, high blood pressure, heart trouble, mood disorders, serious hypoglycemia, diabetes, or any acute physical discomfort, you will have special requirements. You need to be seeing a doctor who knows you are an alcoholic and who understands nutrition. The International College of Applied Nutrition can refer you to a physician and/or nutritionist who can help you refine your health program.

Most alcoholics suffer from some form of digestive problem, such as constipation, colitis, and other disorders involving the intestinal tract. We have created havoc by consistently irritating this area with the poisons in alcohol and drugs. Nutritious foods can help soothe those irritations and stimulate healthy digestion.

We are used to "quick fixes"—drinks, candy bars, pills, caffeine. A healthy body doesn't work that way, with sudden rushes and unpredictable crashes. It travels along at a steady, balanced pace, like the beating of a well-tuned heart. Diet and exercise cannot provide instant relief for nutritional deficiencies, low blood sugar, and physical illnesses and ailments. They provide long-term stability. They require a change in habits and lifestyles.

It is important to eat high-quality foods to help repair tissues and organs and correct the low-blood-sugar problem. Sugar, like alcohol, is an insidious health crippler. It doesn't make us instantly sick. It makes us dependent on chocolate candy, doughnuts, and birthday cakes. It harms us in countless unseen ways.

Our body needs sugar for heat and energy. Normally, sugar is obtained from carbohydrate-rich foods such as grains, vegetables, potatoes, fruits, breads, beans, and corn. The complex carbohydrates are slowly broken down from their long-chain molecules and changed into smaller molecules of absorbable sugar, called glucose, which is ultimately absorbed slowly through the wall of the small intestine. This sugar is then carried to the liver, where it is converted to glycogen and stored as the need arises for muscle action and brain and nerve function. The stored glycogen is converted to a usable form, glucose, and transported by the blood to the areas where it is needed.

When we eat sugar in the form of natural carbohydrates, our blood and tissues usually contain only the amount of sugar needed for their normal function. However, when we drink alcohol, which is absorbed quickly, sometimes through the membranes of the mouth and stomach, a sudden flood of glucose flows into the bloodstream, causing a tremendous strain on the pancreas and liver, as well as on the adrenal and endocrine glands, which are involved in regulating blood-sugar levels.

When we stop drinking, our bodies do not stop craving those sugar rushes. Many of us learn from our doctors and friends in A.A. that those sudden, uncontrollable urges for a drink can be satisfied with a candy bar. In essence, at that point, sugar is saving our lives, eliminating our body's demand for alcohol. Certainly a chocolate bar is less harmful than a shot of scotch, but in the long run continued heavy consumption of sugar will lead us right back to the bottle, where our troubles began.

Your low-blood-sugar (hypoglycemia) symptoms will not disappear immediately, even if you eliminate both alcohol and sugar from your diet. When your sugar level is low, your body will crave glucose to relieve the symptoms of shakiness, fatigue, irritability, depression. Your body signals that it wants something sweet immediately, either sugar or alcohol.

Bringing your blood-sugar level back to an artificial normality relieves your symptoms only temporarily and will cause you to continue this up-and-down cycle. Your body chemistry is distorted; it will take time to bring it back to normal. A diet rich in proteins and natural sugars can begin stabilizing your sugar levels and diminishing your symptoms and cravings. By eating properly, you will be easing your recovery, bolstering your sobriety, and preventing relapses caused by uncontrollable cravings.

THE OPTIMAL NUTRITION PROGRAM

You will find that what you eat in the RRP Program is nutritious and appealing. The frequent meals combined with high-protein snacks will help stabilize your blood-sugar level. Your daily diet will be made up of the four food groups described in the following paragraphs.

Grains, Beans, Seeds, and Nuts. A group of high-quality foods that is often ignored in the United States consists of grains, beans, seeds, and nuts. These foods are the dietary staple in many countries throughout the world. Their nutritional value is greater, and more complete, than in any other single food. When used properly, grains, beans, seeds, and nuts contain nearly all the nutrients you need for tissue repair, maintenance of health, and prevention of disease. In addition, they contain a substance (the germ) that is important for the life, health, and reproductive ability of human beings.

Grains, beans, seeds, and nuts are great natural sources of unsaturated fatty acids, without which health cannot be maintained. They contain lecithin, which is important for the health of the brain, nerves, glands, and arteries. They contain vitamin E and the B-complex vitamins. Vitamin E is important for the protection of your health and acts as defense against premature aging. The B-complex vitamins are necessary in recovery because they protect your body against stress and help regulate your sugar metabolism. If you lack vitamin B, your adrenal glands, which help control blood-sugar levels, can be damaged; this condition is often found to be at the bottom of low-blood-sugar problems.

Grains, seeds, and nuts also contain valuable minerals and trace elements, including magnesium, manganese, iron, zinc, copper, molybdenum, selenium, chromium, fluorine, silicon, potassium, and phosphorus. Sesame seeds are loaded with calcium. Magnesium, zinc, potassium, chromium, and manganese are important because they help regulate sugar metabolism.

What is the best way to eat seeds—fresh or raw? The good news is you can eat them both ways, but will be able to digest some seeds better if you grind them in a seed grinder (available at any health food store for about $16).

You can grind up a combination of seeds and nuts and sprinkle them on fresh fruit for an early-morning breakfast treat. Or sprinkle them on a warm, satisfying bowl of cooked cereal such as buckwheat or oatmeal, and get your grains, seeds, and nuts together. You can add a little butter, top with fresh fruit, and have a breakfast that will energize you for hours. This meal will release high-quality proteins, fatty acids, and slowly put starches (sugars) into your bloodstream.

Seeds are very valuable as sprouts. A few years ago, sprouts were considered "rabbit food," suitable only for health food fanatics. Now they appear on produce shelves in grocery stores, and sprout-growing kits are readily available. Sprouts are excellent in salads, or just eaten by the handful as snacks. Good sources for sprouts include wheat grains, mung beans, alfalfa seeds, and soybeans.

Seeds and nuts are good protein snacks. Soybeans, buckwheat, sesame seeds, pumpkin seeds, almonds, and peanuts contain proteins. These should be a must in your new food program. Learn to carry little bags of seeds and nuts in your pocket or purse (where you used to stash your candy bars), and eat them whenever the signs of low blood sugar appear.

Beans are the greatest single vegetable source of protein. Tofu, which is made from soybeans, is becoming more popular in vegetarian and Oriental cooking, and is rich in proteins. Tofu can be eaten either raw or cooked, works well as a nutritious meat substitute in salads and casseroles, and is good in dressings and desserts.

Vegetables. Vegetables contain extraordinary amounts of minerals, enzymes, and vitamins. They are crucial to health; it is nearly impossible to overdose on their benefits. They can be eaten raw, straight from the garden, or lightly cooked, without destroying their nutrients. It would be ideal if you could have at least one meal a day consisting of a tossed salad full of vegetables.

I admit I was easily bored when I first started adding vegetables to my food plan: I didn't find them very interesting or satisfying. But by reading vegetarian and Oriental cookbooks and browsing through produce stands and health food stores, I discovered many delicious and nutritious foods. Whenever I visited my family in San Francisco, I inevitably ended up in Chinatown, visiting the kitchens of some of the most unusual restaurants I'd ever seen, watching the chefs juggle and blend an amazing array of flavors and textures. I found you could add ginger root and lemon grass to the water when steaming vegetables to give them a delicate, unusual flavor, and learned how to quickly stir-fry a wok full of vegetables with a minimal amount of oil in just a few minutes, creating a satisfying meal. As I experimented and explored, I sometimes went overboard, overcooking the vegetables into an unsightly mush or mixing flavors and colors that clashed unappetizingly. But I also discovered an amazing array of foods and realized how much lighter and energetic I felt when I used vegetables rather than junk foods or meat to satisfy my hunger.

Green vegetables are rich in vitamins and minerals and should be a part of each day's diet. Spinach, peas, beans, and lettuce are great, but expand your tastes by trying asparagus, sprouts, beet greens, collard greens, kale, mustard greens, broccoli, cabbage, and brussels sprouts. Squashes add color and a solid base for casseroles; onions and garlic are indispensable for flavoring. Root vegetables such as carrots, turnips, potatoes, rutabaga, and daikon (a long white radish from Japan now grown in the States) add flavor and crunch when used either cooked or raw.

A vegetable worth mentioning is the avocado, a staple of life on the West Coast. I recommend them highly, either mixed with tomatoes, onions, and chilis into Mexican guacamole, added raw to salads, used as an edible container for fish and chicken salads, or baked in the oven. The avocado rates high on the list of what to include in this new food program. This vegetable is about the only food I am aware of that has perfect nutritional values. It contains protein, fats, carbohydrates, minerals, and vitamins in excellent proportions. But for those concerned about losing weight, be careful; the avocado is loaded with calories. You might want to eat just a half at a time.

Buy fresh vegetables whenever possible, varying your selection with what is in season. Canned and frozen vegetables lack the flavor and nutritional benefits of fresh vegetables. And remember, most vegetables taste as good raw as they do cooked, and contain very few calories. You can munch to your heart's content on carrots, celery, lettuce, and cucumbers and only help your health.

Fruits. Fruits are important because they contain sugar in its natural form. Despite all the damage sugar can cause, it is an essential food. Fruits give your body the sugar it needs, without all the harmful additives in candy. They feed your system with vitamins and minerals and aid digestion. But even fruits must be eaten in moderation, since their sugar can cause your blood sugar to rise rapidly if you eat large amounts.

Some good choices would be sour apples, cherries, strawberries, papaya, grapefruit, lemon, lime, and pineapple. In-season fruits taste best, and their nutrients are at their prime.

Lemons are wonderful for the overworked damaged liver. If you use the juice of half a lemon in the water you drink each day, you will find it can revitalize your liver.

Supplements. Later on in this book, you will learn how to use vitamin and mineral supplements to enhance your nutritional recovery. You will need such supplements less if you start adding natural foods that are rich in nutrients.

Honey helps heal kidney and liver disorders and aids in circulation. It also helps curb sugar cravings, but should be used in moderation—no more than one teaspoon a day. Those who suffer from low blood sugar should keep all sugar intake down. Always make sure that the honey is raw, unrefined, unfiltered, and unheated.

Brewer's yeast is a strong source of an important trace element called chromium. In a recent research project, when rats consumed chromium in the form of brewer's yeast, they metabolized sugar more efficiently.

Since the alcoholic's body has difficulty metabolizing sugar and could be lacking chromium, it is important to increase intake of this element. Chromium is available in small amounts in fish, poultry, beef, whole-grain breads and cereals, cheese, nuts, and dried fruits. However, it is difficult to resolve chromium deprivation simply by eating these foods. By adding brewer's yeast to your diet, you can easily reach the daily recommended dosage of 50 to 100 micrograms of chromium per day.

Many of the people I work with dislike the taste of brewer's yeast, even when it is dissolved in juices or shakes. If you find you dislike the taste or react unpleasantly when you try to take all you need at one time, switch to using brewer's yeast in pill form three times a day. You will discover that if you add brewer's yeast to your new food plan, your sugar cravings decrease and your energy between meals increases.

DANGER ZONES

Inevitably, you will have to eliminate some substances from your diet to get the full benefits from the Recovery/Relapse-Prevention Program. Supplements cannot replace healthy foods; spotty approaches to good nutrition cannot eliminate the harmful effects of unhealthy foods. Ideally, the following substances should never enter your body, but for many of us, that requirement seems impossible to meet. Still, it is possible to avoid dangerous substances when you know what they are, and to approach unhealthy foods with caution. Eventually, the benefits from healthy eating will be so obvious that consuming these unhealthy substances will seem unnecessary.

The *danger zones* is my term for the following categories:

• White sugar and all products made with it: ice cream, pastries, cookies, candies, breakfast cereals, soft drinks, commercially baked breads. I cannot overemphasize the necessity of staying away from all forms of concentrated sugars.
• All other forms of sugar, such as brown, raw, turbinado, and fruit sugar. These should be avoided. Honey can be used, but

only in moderation. You should not use more than a half-teaspoon at a time, with a maximum of one teaspoon a day.

- White flour and everything made with it: bread (you will find that bread sold as brown or whole-grain bread contains white flour—read the labels), packaged breakfast cereals, cookies, pastries, pies, and gravies.
- All soft drinks and so-called juice drinks. Even drinks that are sugar-free should be avoided, because they have artificial flavorings and sweeteners and strong acids that unnecessarily strain your system.
- Excessive amounts of sweet fruit or vegetable juices, even if they are natural and without added sugar. Orange juice, grape juice, apple juice, and carrot juice all contain large amounts of sugar and are harmful when consumed in large amounts.
- All processed, canned, and refined foods, even frozen dinners and breakfast cereals. You should buy only fresh foods, grains, vegetables, and fruits, and make your own meals.
- Too much protein (particularly from meat). This is not advisable, since the digestion required puts a strain on damaged organs. A moderate amount of meat or fish should be included in your meal plans. Do not worry that eating less fish and meat will eliminate protein from your diet. If you follow the whole food plan and increase your consumption of vegetables, beans, seeds, grains, and nuts, you will be getting enough protein. Adding fish or poultry to a few meals each week will give you additional protein without the harmful side effects of other meats.
- Coffee, tea, and caffeine-containing soft drinks, such as colas. Caffeine aggravates the stomach, raises your blood-sugar level, and causes problems with the central nervous system, heart muscles, and respiratory system. It can be difficult to eliminate caffeine from your diet; many people suffer from headaches when they stop drinking coffee. Wean yourself off caffeine gradually.
- Tobacco. It makes us susceptible to many cancers, heart

diseases, and pulmonary disorders. Smoking is an addiction that must be stopped.

CHANGING YOUR EATING HABITS

Most alcoholics have terrible eating habits and almost no rhyme or reason for when to eat, how to eat, and what to eat. Incorporate the following healthy eating habits into your new lifestyle.

* Eat only when you are hungry, but try to eat at regular intervals. Discipline yourself to eat small, nutritious quantities of food three times a day. It is important to eat at scheduled times to help get you back into a disciplined lifestyle. It is imperative to eat a good breakfast.
* Eat slowly in a relaxed atmosphere. When you eat slowly, you will feel satisfied sooner, and you will require less food. Since many recovering alcoholics are overweight, this is important to remember.
* Practice eating less. Overeating is one of the main causes of disease and premature aging. Those who live to be 100 years old aren't overweight. When you eat more than your body requires, you are actually putting a stress on your system with excessive amounts of sugar.

NEW DRINKING HABITS

The final topic of this chapter is new drinking habits. What do you drink? Are you ready for this? *Water!*

Most people entering recovery are dehydrated. Isn't this ironic? Here we were, pouring down fluids, and yet our bodies were starved for water. I know many readers will say, "But I never drink very much water, and I don't think I can start now." But your body needs water to help regulate your kidneys, salivary glands, sweat glands, and intestinal tract. Without water, these organs and glands can literally dry up and cease to function. You must get in the habit of drinking water (at least two and a half quarts daily) to meet the basic water needs.

The best kind of water to drink is natural mineralized water. Much tap water is too polluted to drink safely. Most stores have the kind of water I am recommending.

When fed the proper foods and vitamin supplements combined with exercise, your body can be dramatically restored to health. Your cells can regenerate, toxins can be eliminated, and you can slowly begin the process of healing.

ASSIGNMENTS

1. Create your self-portrait of the healthy, happy person you will be. Hang it beside your current self-portrait.
2. See a doctor, explain your history and symptoms, and be sure you are ready to start the Recovery/Relapse-Prevention Program.
3. Visit produce stands, grocery stores, and health food shops. Become familiar with healthy foods.
4. Clean out your cabinets and refrigerator, discarding all unhealthy foods.

4
Your Nutritional Evaluation

*W*hen I first started working with recovering alcoholics, I gave them a list of foods to avoid and sample menus to use. After a couple of weeks they would seem discouraged, feeling no better. I would ask what they had been eating. Most couldn't remember further back than that day.

Like most of us, they were unaware of their daily diets. Maybe they felt nagging guilt about eating too much sugar or junk food, but they had no idea just how much they were eating, what they were eating, or why they ate when they did. Before they could possibly change their eating habits, they had to know what those habits were. With that knowledge, they succeeded in changing their diets. Discouragement disappeared. Encouragement was easy, because they were feeling great.

Spend a week getting to know yourself and your attitudes toward food and eating before you plunge into the Recovery/ Relapse-Prevention Program.

YOUR MEASUREMENT CHART

To find out how your nutritional and fitness programs change your body, weigh and measure yourself now. Fill in your measurements on the Measurement Chart on page 182. If you want to lose (or gain) weight and inches, fill in the goal sections and weigh and measure yourself every two weeks. Fill in your short- and long-term goals, using new copies of the chart as you progress. Combine diet with your exercise program to firm up problem areas, and use a scale and measuring tape to chart your progress. Chapter 6 has more suggestions for weight loss, based on healthful principles.

YOUR SEVEN-DAY DIET DIARY

You *must* complete your Daily Diet Diary before your new eating program starts. It will help you evaluate your eating patterns.

The Daily Diet Diary in Appendix A (page 183) should be nearby at all times during your diary week. Carry one chart each day. You can transfer this chart to a notebook or index cards, or jot down what and why you eat during the day and transfer the information to the chart at night. This gives you a chance to review your day and think a little more about why you eat.

In the appropriate columns, write down everything you eat and drink. You may be surprised, even alarmed, at the length of the lists and the enormous amounts of sugar you are consuming. This is normal, believe me.

You are using this diary to learn what you eat. Don't make any drastic changes while observing yourself. Eat what you normally do, and be honest enough to write everything down. Imagine how proud you will be a month from now when you look back at this chart and remember how you felt and looked.

In the middle column, record situations and moods; this is central to your recovery. You may find that you eat for the same reasons you used to drink, and may be continuing harmful habits out of boredom, lack of motivation, loss of incentive, or simply to "stuff your feelings." By filling in this column honestly, you will uncover the reasons you eat what and when you do. What makes you sit down and eat? Is it habit (12:00 noon = lunchtime), stress, anger, loneliness? Have you ever wondered about that? Now is your time to find out.

It is important to stick with your diary for the full seven days, in order to get a reliable pattern. Your diary should highlight the factors that consistently determine the way you eat. These discoveries will clarify your path to success. Combine your diet with a restructured lifestyle. Release your emotions and stress in healthy ways, using the Recovery/Relapse-Prevention Fitness Program in Part Two.

ASSIGNMENTS

1. Weigh and measure yourself, and fill in the blanks on your Measurement Chart.
2. Begin and complete your Daily Diet Diary.

5
Your Daily Diet

Your Daily Diet Diary is a chart of your past and a tool you can use throughout the Recovery/Relapse-Prevention Program. Once you have completed it, you are aware of your eating preferences and habits. You are now ready to embark on a path to your new eating program for recovery, relapse prevention, and health.

GETTING STARTED

Most recovering alcoholics discover they have a sugar problem. Even though you now know that sugar is your enemy, it will take an ongoing effort to eliminate it from your diet. It's possible that many of the foods you usually eat contain sugar. They will have to be replaced. For now, forget they exist, and experiment with healthy, nutritious foods. Your choices will be different, unusual, unlike your current favorite foods. They may seem limited, but may also open a whole menu of tastes you have never experienced. Experiment with the full range of foods included in your new

41

nutritional plan, and with spices, herbs, and recipes. Consider yourself to be on a culinary adventure.

Begin by following the Seven-Day Menu Plan in Appendix A (pages 184–87) exactly as it is, using the simplest foods: raw and cooked vegetables, meats and fish broiled or baked, raw fruit for desserts, milk, nuts, or cheese for snacks. After your first week, start using one new recipe every day. After you find a recipe you enjoy, repeat it, then try a new one. Prepare extra portions of favorite recipes and freeze them. Rotate new foods with your favorites so you won't become bored.

Use all kinds of vegetables. Try serving a green and red vegetable at each meal. Once a week, buy a new vegetable you rarely eat. Try it two or three different ways to see if you can find a way you like.

Experiment with new sources of protein, cutting down on your meat intake. If you don't like fish, try it in other forms—say, clam chowder or shrimp salad. Be good to yourself once a week and make a full-course meal, including an extra-special dessert. Stay away from restaurants until you catch on to this food program.

As your food choices and eating habits change, you will find that the urge for carbohydrates and sugar disappears.

Finally, remember that the most important by-product of this program is a renewed feeling of health. If you follow the program carefully, you will feel energy and a sense of well-being you thought had become a thing of the past. Your chances of relapse will decrease significantly.

Study the Food Chart in Appendix A (pages 188–89) to determine what you can and cannot eat. Use it as your guide throughout your menu planning, making notes on your likes and dislikes, and adding new options as you find them.

TIPS FOR SUCCESS

So many of the people I have worked with (including myself) never had a regular schedule for eating. But to experience real control over what you eat and not be driven to eat foolishly when you get ravenously hungry, you must eat at regular times each day. When you skip meals, your blood-sugar level will plunge, and you may head to the nearest candy rack (or drink or drug) for that quick pick-me-up.

Eat snacks between meals. Stick with those on your snack list.

The best time to get started is over the weekend. Use this time to do your menu planning and shopping (not when you're hungry). The Seven-Day Menu Plan will be your initial blueprint.

Make your own menu forms for following weeks, varying the selections from week 1. Stick with the things you liked. Once you follow the Seven-Day Menu Plan, you will get the hang of how your new eating program works.

Start now, at week 1, to follow this program as closely as you possibly can. Buy fresh fruits, vegetables, fish, and meat. Find shops that sell whole-wheat bread and whole-wheat pasta (most supermarkets and health food stores stock them), and try to follow the recipes where they are given.

This program is healthy and rich in complex carbohydrates, low in refined carbohydrates and fat, moderate in protein and high in fresh fruits and vegetables, often raw, for maximum nutritional value. Sugar is obsolete.

Once you get familiar with this program, you will find it very flexible. When you fully comprehend the amounts of complex carbohydrates, protein, and fat outlined in the box below, it will be

---

DAILY FOOD REQUIREMENT

Based on the amount of total food energy—2,500 calories for men and 2,000 calories for women—your daily food requirements should consist of the following approximate percentages:

protein	15–25%
complex carbohydrates	55–65%
fats	10–25%

smooth sailing for you. The only thing you will have to plan ahead of time will be your Survival Kit (described in Appendix A, page 190) to get you through sugar cravings and low-energy periods.

Whether you cook for yourself or a family, eat on the run, or eat a lot in restaurants, these rules will help you put together the proper meal:

- Make your breakfast full of fruits and whole grains, such as a bran muffin with farmer's cheese and sliced apples. You can follow the three breakfast choices and interchange them during the week.
- Think of grains first. Don't think, "What am I going to cook with my chicken?" Once you have decided on a starch, then choose a vegetable and fruit to complete the complex-carbohydrate group.
- Limit intake of high-quality protein (meat, poultry, eggs, and cheese). Eaten in small quantities, they will meet your daily requirements.
- Rely on natural herbs and spices to flavor your food and replace gooey sauces and dressings you don't need.
- Spruce up your main meals and make them enticing. Add bright slices of tomatoes, green-pepper strips, sliced radishes, melon curls, sprigs of parsley, or sliced apples.
- If you have to eat out, ask for simply prepared meat and fish (stay away from rich sauces), unbuttered vegetables, salads with little dressing, fresh fruit instead of heavy desserts.
- Drink at least six to eight glasses of water a day (bottled or tap) and decaffeinated herbal teas. Drink decaffeinated coffee, and experiment with the huge range of herbal teas that are now available. You will find they have a calming or stimulating effect, depending on your choice, and taste delicious.

You are now ready to start your food program and are on your way to regaining your health and vitality.

ASSIGNMENTS

1. Consult the Seven-Day Menu Plan and Food Chart. Make a shopping list.
2. Buy all the groceries you need, but only enough fresh vegetables and fruit for the first few days. Replenish your stock according to your taste preferences.
3. Follow your Seven-Day Menu Plan faithfully. Jot notes to yourself on the menus, marking the items you particularly like or dislike.
4. Assemble your Survival Kit in a small cooler or lunch box and carry it with you. Stock your office with fruit, vegetables, and healthy snacks.

6
Weight Control

*I*rene became my client shortly after leaving a recovery house, where she had successfully completed a three-month stay. "I want to lose 20 pounds," she said over and over. "I want to lose 20 pounds."

I outlined a food program and a moderate walking program to start her off. I told her it was important to eat three meals a day and lose a maximum of two pounds a week. We set a target date for her target weight, allowing 10 weeks for her to lose those 20 pounds. We met once every two weeks to monitor her progress.

She lost seven pounds in the first two weeks. I thought that was quite a bit, but assumed that most of it was water loss. I did not see her again until the end of the fourth week. I noticed how gaunt and fatigued she looked. I got her on the scale right away, and she had lost 12 more pounds. Nineteen pounds altogether in only four weeks!

She beamed with pride and said the real, elegant, fragile Irene had emerged and was here to stay.

She was elated. I was upset. I told her that she had lost the weight too quickly, which was dangerous. Just how had she lost this weight? I knew it wasn't on my program.

SWITCHING OBSESSIONS

Irene told me she didn't follow the food program I had given her. She nearly starved herself the first two weeks, thus losing the initial seven pounds. Then she went on an "official diet" that had her eating nothing but fish, chicken, eggs, and farmer's cheese. She weighed herself three times a day, declined all invitations that included eating, and crossed the street to avoid passing the bakery. "Gorging" on a potato with dinner one night meant eating nothing but lettuce and a boiled egg the next day. And sometimes, she said, "I'd catch myself looking at people at A.A. meetings, and looking at their bulges of fat. Gloating to myself. I know that wasn't very nice."

Irene had let her addictive behavior take over. In essence, all she had done was to switch her addiction from alcohol to food. Irene, like many recovering alcoholics, had not yet learned to free herself from compulsions and obsessions. Her approach to food was fraught with emotional pitfalls.

If we allow ourselves to become obsessed with fanatical dieting, we are actually distorting our perceptions. Every little slip of the fork seems like a major moral collapse. We get emotional, distracted, agitated. Sobriety, with all the concerns and changes surrounding that major change in our lives, becomes more and more difficult. We adopt an on-the-wagon/off-the-wagon mentality.

I told Irene she needed to start eating three nutritious meals a day and to see her physician immediately. She shut me out. I tried calling her to set up another appointment, but she was always "overcommitted." Two months later, during one of my weekly calls, she agreed to get together with me. I was shocked when I saw her. She had gained 28 pounds. Her weight had zoomed up to a new high.

Irene was once again overweight and depressed. She was tired of it all, she said, tired of the wild weight swings up and down, tired of the search for new diets, tired of the constant obsession with food. Her life in sobriety was getting too busy to allow such indulgence.

A DIFFERENT APPROACH

Irene agreed to follow my program, and quit eating obsessively. She learned the basics of nutrition, and developed a working knowledge of portion sizes. She bought a small postage scale, measuring cups, and measuring spoons. She shopped for groceries with portions in mind, and found that if she used premeasured meat or fish from the store, and cooked it, there would usually be a one-ounce loss.

Irene was now ready to exercise. She joined the health club where I work as a private trainer and followed a beginner's program of weight training, aerobic-dance classes, and daily morning walks.

Irene has been following her nutrition and fitness program for two years now, and it has served her body well. She reached her ideal weight of 120 pounds, losing 30 pounds in one year. She learned to maintain her weight by continuing to exercise regularly and eating three nutritious meals a day.

Like Irene, very few of my clients are truly obese. Most want to lose five to twenty pounds. And like Irene, most are obsessive about what they eat.

Food, like alcohol and drugs, can control your life. If you are in A.A., you know it takes a tremendous personal and spiritual investment to conquer any addiction. Overeaters Anonymous gives you those skills and is an invaluable resource for those trying to control their eating habits. Attend a few O.A. meetings as you begin your nutrition and fitness program. The support, encouragement, and understanding you will receive from other O.A. members will help you change your attitudes toward food and toward your body.

The Recovery/Relapse-Prevention Program is not a diet. It is a dietary plan geared toward health and the elimination of cravings for sugar and alcohol. But the basics of this program are the same as the basics of any reputable diet. With a few adjustments to the dietary plan, you can begin losing weight in a sensible, steady manner, avoiding the cravings, binges, fasts, and fads that have kept you in the diet trap.

When you finish reading this book, you will understand the foods that nourish your body and the wisdom of taking in a wide range of foods from all categories—grains, dairy products, fruit and vegetables, and meat, chicken, and fish. It's a mental attitude that accepts eating as a pleasurable experience to be fitted comfortably into your life. The right frame of mind will keep your life from being bound to food or the avoidance of it.

Certain facets of the RRP Program will be particularly helpful to those who want to lose weight and keep the pounds off. By understanding the following concepts, you can learn to control your eating and your weight for life.

METABOLISM

Crash diets allow you to lose more weight in less time than sound nutritional programs do. The problem is, you are losing water, not fat. You are not taking responsibility for your body. You are looking for a quick fix, even if it means depriving yourself of food, energy, and nutrition. When this attitude toward weight loss persists, the urge to eat wins out, and the pounds return. You are setting yourself up for a possible relapse into drugs and alcohol.

It is important for you to understand an internal mechanism called the *setpoint*. This mechanism drives the body to maintain a particular level of body fat. In a practical sense, this is the body weight you maintain when not counting calories.

Everyone has different setpoint factors. Drugs like amphetamines and nicotine lower the setpoint, while dieting has no effect. Each time you manage to reduce your fat level below your natural setpoint, the body makes internal adjustments to reverse this change and conserve body fat.

The *metabolic rate* greatly affects how the body burns calories. When you diet, your metabolic rate actually decreases to protect your body against starvation. The body burns less fat because it is reacting to a reduction in calories. If you were actually starving, this mechanism would save your life. When you are dieting, it prevents you from losing weight. The resting metabolic rate in severe dieting can be lowered as much as 45 percent.

Most overweight people diet in spurts, trying the latest fad, giving up when the pounds just will not come off. Each time you diet, the metabolic rate adjusts to the decrease in calories by slowing down. These adjustments conserve energy and cause your diet to become progressively less effective.

How can you adjust your setpoint and metabolic rate so you can lose weight safely and effectively? By exercising on a daily basis. The only way to achieve long-lasting success in controlling your weight is to restructure your lifestyle so that vigorous exercise becomes an important, integral part of your daily routine.

Regular exercise keeps the metabolic rate at normally high levels, develops the body's lean tissues and uses up fat, and adjusts your appetite-control level so you eat what you need.

EXERCISE

If you are interested in losing weight, you must face one fact. No one can wave a magic wand and command the fat to disappear. There is no magical secret to losing weight. The clear and simple truth is that the fewer calories you consume and conserve and the more calories you burn, the more weight you will lose. The body's metabolism requires a comprehensive approach to weight loss. Eat fewer calories and exercise consistently, and you *will* lose weight.

Consistent exercise also helps the body regulate its need for food. When you diet and exercise sporadically, with little consistency, your body no longer knows how much food to demand. As a result, you may eat more than you need. In fact, an extremely sedentary lifestyle may be so abnormal that you overeat as a form of stimulation.

Exercise doesn't have to be strenuous or boring. Take the attitude that you can keep your body fit by learning to play. Riding a bike, roller-skating, swimming, and hiking are just a few of the enjoyable activities to choose from.

Start off slowly, listen to your body, and have fun. Let that little boy or little girl out, and learn to play.

SUGAR

When you eliminate sugar from your diet, you automatically reduce your caloric intake. Your blood-sugar level is your key to controlling your weight. You can control your weight successfully when you eat basic foods on a schedule that allows your blood-sugar level to remain in a normal state.

NUTRITIONAL FOODS

Many people think that a weight-control program is made up of boring food, self-denial, deprivation, and guilt. You may have been this route before.

I explain to my clients that they don't have to think this way. The best way to get a grip on the business of weight once and forever is to eat *balanced* meals made up of a wide variety of foods, even including a little fettucine Alfredo or a slice of pumpkin pie now and then. You can try new recipes, serve attractive foods, go out to restaurants and still stay slim.

WEIGHT-LOSS TIPS

Before you start changing your eating and exercise habits, you must get a complete physical checkup. Your doctor may recommend that you have a glucose-tolerance test (a test that assesses your body's sugar-regulating mechanisms) or an EKG stress test to determine how your cardiovascular system is functioning. Be sure that any medical problems that might prevent you from starting a diet/exercise program are taken into consideration, and ask your doctor to help adapt this program to your needs.

Be realistic about the amount of weight you need to lose. Refer to the Standard Weight Table on page 53 to determine your ideal weight, and use that as your goal.

Recovery teaches us to live in the present. We are urged to give up our "old ideas." You can apply these same principles to your new eating and fitness program.

The RRP Program is based on an integrated approach. It offers you the chance to:

- Lose weight
- Begin exercising toward physical fitness
- Learn basic principles of good nutrition
- Learn how to apply them, implementing a basic diet designed for optimum nutritional health

Be sure to complete the Daily Diet Diary from Chapter 4, and continue keeping a daily record of what you eat and how you feel. You may begin to see that you eat for emotional reasons rather than to curb your hunger. Once you understand your eating behaviors, you will be better able to stabilize your eating.

A realistic weight-loss goal is one to two pounds a week. To lose one pound of fat, you must reduce your food intake by 3,500 calories, or burn off the equivalent of 3,500 calories through exercise. If a person normally eats 2,500 calories a day and reduces that intake to 1,500 calories a day, he or she will lose two pounds a week.

Knowing how to cut calories and eating a well-balanced diet are the only sure ways to stay healthy while losing weight and keeping it off permanently. Eating a variety from all food groups is a good place to start. Ideally, you should eat a minimum number of

STANDARD WEIGHT TABLE

Men

Height	Small	Medium	Large
5'2"	128–134	131–141	138–150
5'3"	130–136	133–143	140–153
5'4"	132–138	135–145	142–156
5'5"	134–140	137–148	144–160
5'6"	136–142	139–151	146–164
5'7"	138–145	142–154	149–168
5'8"	140–148	145–157	152–172
5'9"	142–151	148–160	155–176
5'10"	144–154	151–163	158–180
5'11"	146–157	154–166	161–184
6'0"	149–160	157–170	164–188
6'1"	152–164	160–174	168–192
6'2"	155–168	164–178	172–197
6'3"	158–172	167–182	176–202
6'4"	164–176	171–187	181–207

Women

Height	Small	Medium	Large
4'10"	102–111	109–121	118–131
4'11"	103–113	111–123	120–134
5'0"	104–115	113–125	122–137
5'1"	106–118	115–129	125–140
5'2"	108–121	118–132	128–143
5'3"	111–124	121–135	131–147
5'4"	114–127	124–138	134–151
5'5"	117–130	127–141	137–155
5'6"	120–133	130–144	140–159
5'7"	123–136	133–147	143–163
5'8"	126–139	136–150	146–167
5'9"	129–142	139–153	149–170
5'10"	132–145	142–156	152–173
5'11"	135–148	145–159	155–176
6'0"	138–151	148–162	158–179

These tables were published in 1983 by the Metropolitan Life Insurance Company. All heights are with shoes: men's weights include 5 and women's include 3 pounds of indoor clothing.

portions in each of these food groups every day. If you follow these guidelines, you will get the proper nutrients your body needs.

Food Group	Portions/Day	Servings/Portion
Cereal/grain	4	{ 1 slice bread { ½ cup cereal or pasta
Fruit/vegetable	3–5	½ cup
Meat/protein	2	3 ounces
Milk/dairy	2	1 cup

The sample Seven-Day Menu Plan from Chapter 5 will help you get started. As you become accustomed to the Food Chart on pages 188–89, you will be able to plan nutritious, low-calorie meals based on your tastes. By combining this plan with exercise, you will soon begin losing weight.

The importance of developing good eating habits goes beyond just weight control. Foods that are low in calories are also generally those that decrease the risk of developing heart disease and cancer. A healthy diet is one that includes foods that are low in saturated fat, cholesterol, salt, and refined sugar, and high in fiber, vitamins, and minerals.

Restructuring your meals to supply calories when they will be used most effectively will speed the burning of fat. You are going to be eating three meals a day that correspond with your body's energy needs:

• Fuel up at breakfast.
• Replenish at lunch.
• Maintain at dinner.

Certain foods like honey, sprouts, and whole grains carry extra energy nutrients. These are all included in the menu plan. Don't forget to take your vitamin/mineral supplements to further bolster energy.

Changing habits, even poor ones, can be difficult. It requires a great deal of patience, commitment, faith, and willingness. It will be easier if you concentrate on the benefits and use a support system like O.A.

Remember to take this change one day at a time. Don't think of tomorrow, a week, a month, or a lifetime. Concentrate on your change for today, and all the tomorrows will be taken care of.

Reward yourself not only for losing pounds, but also for sticking with your diet and exercise program. You may be accustomed to food rewards; work at finding other things that give you pleasure—new clothes, a bouquet of flowers, tickets to a sporting or cultural event, a trip to show off your new body to an old friend.

Finally, be patient with yourself. You are embarking on a new food regimen, and your body will be confused. You may also feel psychologically confused and uncomfortable as you try to eliminate familiar patterns and foods. Don't panic if you make mistakes in the beginning.

Staying slim, if you are accustomed to being overweight, need not be a constant battle. The secret of a successful weight-control program is its ability to help you keep the pounds off once you have reached your desired weight. The RRP Program helps you do just that, because it allows you to gradually integrate healthy eating and exercise habits into your life. If you decide that you want to live your life in a lean, attractive body, you can. Remember, you alone control what and how much you eat and how active you are. If you eat right and keep physically active, you will control your weight, stay trim, and be a few steps ahead on your path to safe and sane sobriety.

ASSIGNMENTS

1. Assemble your Measurement Chart, your Seven-Day Diet Diary, the Seven-Day Menu Plan, and your self-portraits in a notebook.
2. Study your completed Seven-Day Diet Diary from Chapter 4, comparing it to the Seven-Day Menu Plan in Chapter 5.
3. Make your own personalized Food Chart, including the foods from your diet diary that are in both the Eat Freely and the Eat Sparingly columns. Try to make your Eat Freely column longer than your Eat Sparingly column.
4. Continue recording each day's consumption as you learn to adapt your diet.

7
Supplements for Health

*W*hen I discovered how to use nutritional supplements (vitamins and minerals), I started feeling better than I had in years. I met with biochemists and nutritionists and read everything I could find on using nutritional supplements to combat the damage from drugs and alcohol. Gradually I developed a nutritional program, learning what supplements to use, what dosages to take, and when to take them.

At first, I wondered how a pill or powder could alter my sugar cravings, reduce my stress, and increase my energy. I didn't have to wonder for long. In just weeks I noticed a radical change in my health. I found I had a new zest for life. Nutritional supplements became an integral part of my healing process, as important as any other aspect of my recovery plan.

Most of my clients like this part of their program. I'm sure you know why. We were all a bunch of pill poppers and could readily comprehend the idea of taking pills that were *good* for us. Plus, we were adding something new to our lives, not trying to get rid of some old bad habit.

Naturally, some of us went overboard with our supplements, gleefully thinking that these pills could replace good nutrition, that we could continue gorging on junk food as long as we took our vitamins every day. *Vitamins and minerals are not substitutes for good nutrition. They are supplements.* Nothing can replace the benefits of healthful foods. There is no sense in taking supplements if you are not eating the right foods.

Conventional programs for treating drug and alcohol abuse view those in recovery as being healthy. The concept is that once you stop drinking and drugging, your nutritional deficits will be resolved and your body will return to a healthy state. In reality, the opposite is true. Our nutritional needs remain critical long after we stop abusing drugs and alcohol.

VITAMIN TREATMENT METHODS

The first research on vitamin treatment methods that I discovered was performed by Doctors Hoffer and Oswold. Thirty years ago, when trying to rehabilitate alcoholics, they used large doses of vitamin B_3 along with more limited doses of other vitamins and minerals. They also used a controlled diet, eliminating all caffeine and sugar.

The study showed that whenever this treatment was used, the results were significantly better than those from more conventional treatment methods. Recovery rates of 80 percent were reported, in contrast to the 70 percent relapse rates reported for conventional treatment methods.

This study and the other information in this book should make it obvious that physical recovery depends on the quality of nutrition. The RRP Program is geared toward resolving nutritional deficiencies. It is not megavitamin therapy or some sort of miraculous cure. It is a method of gradually adapting your lifestyle and habits into a healthier form, designed to help heal the special physical problems incurred by alcohol and drug abuse. By supplementing your food plan with the necessary vitamins and minerals, you are helping your body function properly and ward off disease.

THE ROLE OF VITAMINS AND MINERALS

Do not expect vitamins and minerals to be a cure-all. They can only help rectify your nutritional and physical deficiencies. Vitamins help increase the rate of chemical reactions that occur in the body. A person in good health who eats a well-balanced, nutritional diet does not need supplements, but you do need them at first to help your body return to a healthy state. Minerals help regulate the body's fluids and balance of chemicals. A deficit of certain vitamins and minerals can lead to serious diseases. Vitamins and minerals alone cannot cure chronic physical ailments. If you are feeling unwell, you should see a doctor and go over your nutritional program with him or her.

Sometimes it takes a few weeks to feel the effects of your nutritional supplement program, though I have had a few clients who report significant changes in only one week. For example, the chromium, glutamine, and magnesium supplements had an immediate effect on their craving for sweets.

Since everyone's body is unique in size, shape, and biochemical makeup, nutritional needs differ. Therefore, vitamin and mineral dosages must be tailored to your individual needs. You can determine your needs by experimenting with dosages, or visit a nutritionist or doctor who can evaluate your needs.

A PLAN WITH THE BASICS

The program outlined here provides the basics, a starting point for your nutritional rehabilitation. As you read through the Vitamin Summary and the Mineral Summary in Appendix A (pages 192–209), use the form on pages 210–11 to jot down the supplements you think your body needs, paying close attention to the foods you can eat to help bolster your intake of vitamins and minerals. As you begin taking supplemental vitamins and minerals, follow the recommended dosages and see how your body reacts. All supplements should be taken with meals. Multivitamins are best when taken with breakfast; others may go down more easily if the dosage is divided throughout the day.

60   *Staying* SOBER

The vitamin and mineral charts reproduced in Appendix A were initially printed in *Eating Right to Live Sober* by Katherine Ketcham and L. Ann Mueller, M.D., published by Signet Books. This book is an excellent resource for those who are seriously interested in learning about their bodies' nutritional needs.

ASSIGNMENTS

1. Complete your personalized Vitamin and Mineral List.
2. Shop for vitamins and minerals. Store in refrigerator or other cool, dark place.
3. Begin taking the minimum dosages.
4. Record your reactions.
5. Increase or decrease dosages as needed.
6. Consult with a physician or nutritionist for a complete nutritional evaluation.

PART II
FITNESS

The journey of a thousand miles
Must begin with a single step.

LAO-TZU

8
Low-Level Fitness
Equals Low-Level Health

Most alcoholics who enter recovery are in the middle to late stages of alcoholism. Damage to our livers, central nervous systems, and vital organs is almost certain. No wonder our physical strength is impaired and our resistance to disease is lowered. Our reasoning, perception, memory, and judgment are affected. Our mental and emotional stability is questionable. Most of us have some form of sugar-regulating disorder. We suffer from malnutrition. These conditions, if not corrected, will keep us from enjoying a complete, full life.

If our disease is not treated as a physical disease and we relapse, alcohol will go on to destroy our hearts, brains, stomachs, lungs, and kidneys. If one of these organs fails, we most assuredly will die sooner than we otherwise must. If you are a recovering alcoholic who still smokes, drinks a lot of coffee, and consumes a great deal of sugar, your risks for heart failure and cancer are multiplied.

I've heard a lot of angry people say, "I can't quit smoking and give up sugar, coffee, and alcohol at the same time—I'll go nuts!" I haven't had enough time to stop and give them a two-hour lecture

63

on why these things are so important to give up. I hope they will understand more when they read this book.

Alcohol's effect on the heart is a major cause of death in alcoholism. It has been shown that alcohol and alcohol toxicity affect the cell membranes in the heart muscle, which changes its shape and functioning. Many alcoholics suffer from high blood pressure as well as cardiac arrhythmia (irregular heartbeat).

If you have heart problems, you can still live a normal, healthy life, but you must be willing to go to any lengths to enjoy it. You must give up coffee drinking, smoking, and poor eating habits. You owe it to yourself and your family and friends. If you cared enough to give up alcohol, it only makes sense to give up the rest. Take this book to your doctor and discuss your nutritional and fitness needs.

CHANGES IN THE LIVER

I cut up a cadaver as part of my training in physical education. I will never forget the size of the liver. It was the biggest organ in the body. It is behind the rib cage on the right side and cannot be felt from outside. The liver can get very swollen and painful.

Too much alcohol in your system over a long period of time builds fat in the liver. Excess fat circulates in your bloodstream, affecting the capillaries and circulation and reducing the oxygen to the brain cells. A fatty liver can cause the liver cells to die. As each cell is injured, the fatty deposits expand and cause the liver to swell. When I see a beer-guzzling person with a large gut, I can just imagine what his liver looks like.

The next stage is alcoholic hepatitis, then cirrhosis of the liver. At this point the liver is clogged up and can't function. The blood vessels become constricted and can hemorrhage, causing death. At this stage, the liver's ability to detoxify poisons is hindered. Ammonia can build up in the blood stream, which can also cause death. Another poison is bilirubin, which causes yellowing of the skin (jaundice).

If you continue to drink or relapse into these final stages, death awaits you. If you stop drinking, there is hope, because the liver has extraordinary recuperative powers. The liver can be amazingly transformed with the proper care. If you eliminate alcohol and cigarettes, eat the right food and supplements, rest and slowly start to exercise, the liver will do all it can to regenerate itself.

OTHER CHANGES

Alcohol also affects the lining of the stomach, leading to gastritis and ulcers. Alcohol interferes with the body's immune system, resulting in susceptibility to respiratory infections. Tuberculosis, chronic bronchitis, emphysema, and lung abscesses are prevalent. Pneumonia is a common cause of death for alcoholics.

There is still a great deal of research going on in the area of cancer and its relationship to alcohol. Alcoholics who smoke face the possibility of tar buildup causing cancers of the mouth, lungs, and esophagus.

As previously described, malnutrition is a by-product of alcoholism. If this goes unchecked, mental and physical disorders and death will follow.

THE IMPORTANCE OF PHYSICAL FITNESS

I won't belabor the debilitating effects of alcohol and drugs any longer. But I will repeat again and again that you can overcome much of the damage and return your body to a healthy, energetic state. Thus far, you have learned various ways to start rebuilding your health with nutritional foods and supplements. Now you will learn the importance of physical fitness.

Lack of regular vigorous physical activity contributes to overweight and the deterioration of the circulatory system, which results in cardiovascular and coronary disease. Inadequate circulation of the blood prevents vital food elements from being sufficiently distributed throughout the body. This leads to fatigue and low endurance.

When we get out of shape, we become susceptible to minor ailments, which can lead to more serious illnesses. Research has shown that the probability of early death is high for people who exhibit a poor fitness profile at an early age.

The absence of physical ailments is a critical part of health, but not all of it. A broken leg certainly can hamper the quality of your life, but you can still be relatively healthy. On the other hand, a severely depressed person can have all parts of the body in perfect working order and be so unhealthy as to risk his or her own life.

Most communicable diseases have been controlled by modern medicine. Vulnerability to disease is thought to be related to factors including the physical and mental hazards that fill our environment: cancer-causing substances, stress, poor nutrition, little or no exercise. Modern-day technology has altered most occupations and modes of transportation. We are required to spend less energy in our everyday activities. Most of us have adopted sedentary lifestyles, which contribute to ill health.

EVERYDAY DECISIONS

Everyday decisions have an enormous impact on our health. We have decided to quit drinking and using drugs. That is our first step toward taking responsibility for our health. Some of us decide to enter a treatment center. We become members of Alcoholics Anonymous or Narcotics Anonymous. Our next step is to take responsibility for restoring our bodies to health.

We make decisions every day concerning what to eat, whether to smoke or drink coffee, when to exercise, and how to cope with stressful situations. Beyond these issues, we decide when to seek medical, psychological, or dental care. We decide what to tell our doctors, and whether we will follow their advice. The entire process of maintaining or restoring our health depends on our decisions. Health cannot be rebuilt and maintained without our conscious involvement. The first thing we must do is to face the fact that there are no magic cures or shortcuts to regaining our health.

WHAT TO EXPECT

It will take about 12 weeks of hard work for you to regain your physical fitness. It could be the hardest work you have done in a long time. But the benefits (explained in the next chapter) will be worth it. You must be motivated and ready to make a commitment now. Your life and your health depend upon this commitment.

Vitality and a genuine zest for life come from good circulation of the blood; strong, coordinated muscles; and resistance to disease and chronic ailments. You can have all this and more if you participate in a systematic physical fitness program.

Bob E., an A.A. circuit speaker with 24 years of sobriety, offers this testimony about his journey to fitness and health:

"I get more emotional now when I talk about health than I do when talking about recovering from dying, because I have been recovering from dying for 22 years. Health is more recent. Recovery is spiritual, physical, mental, and emotional. I had to deal with the mental and emotional before I got enough self-esteem to work on the physical." Bob now exercises and meditates for an hour and a half every morning of the week but one.

"For those of you who are over 25 and thinking of starting this, I want you to know that you have to be really patient. It took me nine months to be able to do a normal sit-up.

"My normal way of doing something is to take on so much I can't do it. Then, rather than eliminate a couple of things, I eliminate all and go away feeling worthless. That is so lethal.

"The energy we put into keeping the spirit down is incredible. I keep the spirit down because I am afraid of the spirit. I keep the spirit down because I was raised by alcoholics who kept the spirit down. They kept the child down. They made him shut up, sit still, get in the corner, stay out of the way, and keep peace at all costs.

"Now, at 50, I am looking forward to improved health, to improved mental and emotional attitudes, to improved self-esteem. I am looking forward."

Bob E. talks a lot about other people he knows who are actively working at becoming healthy, fit, and happy. Their stories, and those I hear from my clients, have basic similarities. They all end with changes in the quality of their sobriety and recovery. They all learned how to become healthy by changing their nutrition, exercising their bodies, and learning to calm their minds and emotions.

9
Optimal Fitness Equals Optimal Health

*W*hat is a good definition of the word *fitness*? Some people think a physically fit person must look like a body builder and excel in gymnastics, swimming, aerobic dancing, or baseball. In truth, an individual who is physically fit usually looks like the rest of us, because much of fitness is inside the body. Fitness means you can be free from sickness and have a positive mental attitude.

The American Association of Physical Health, Exercise and Recreation (AAPHER) describes fitness as "that state which characterizes the degree to which the person is able to function." The association lists the seven components of fitness, all of which are related to each other and are mutually interdependent. These are:

1. Optimum organic health consistent with heredity and the application of present health knowledge
2. Sufficient coordination, strength, and vitality to meet emergencies as well as the requirements for daily living

69

3. Emotional stability to meet the stresses and strains of modern life
4. Social consciousness and adaptability with respect to the requirements of group living
5. Sufficient knowledge and insight to make suitable decisions and arrive at feasible solutions to problems
6. Attitudes, values, and skills that stimulate satisfactory participation in a full range of daily activities
7. Spiritual and moral qualities that contribute to the fullest measure of living in a pluralistic society

This list highlights the fact that we must integrate the physical, mental, and spiritual philosophy in our recovery to restore our bodies to this accepted definition of fitness. To evaluate health, we have to look at the human organism as an integrated whole. Physical health doesn't start below the neck, and mental health above it. The mind and body are integrated in a way that is intimate and complex. A sick body increases the stress on a healthy mind. A sick mind debilitates the body.

EXERCISE AND HEALTH

The psychological and physical effects of a consistent exercise program include the following:

• Exercise allows the muscles, lungs, and heart to overcome the unhealthy effects of a sedentary lifestyle and alcoholism and drug abuse.
• Exercise reduces the resting and aerobic heart rate, increases the quality and quantity of the blood pumped to the heart, increases the size of the heart muscle, and increases the strength of the heart muscle's contractions. The heart pumps more efficiently, thus increasing the circulation of the blood to vital organs.
• The increased efficiency of the circulatory system improves

skin tone by helping the skin eliminate impurities.

- Exercise reduces resting blood pressure and lessens the potential for hardening of the arteries.
- Exercise increases the lungs' functional capacity, allowing them to exchange oxygen and carbon dioxide more quickly.
- The body's metabolic rate increases with exercise, increasing energy and burning calories more efficiently.
- The bones, joints, ligaments, and muscles strengthen, reducing the likelihood of injuries and physical deterioration.
- Coordination, balance, posture, endurance, and flexibility increase, improving appearance and attitude and reducing the opportunities for injury.
- Exercise can help you quit smoking. I haven't stressed the need to eliminate tobacco from your lifestyle, because we all get discouraged when we think we have to "give up" too much too soon. But you may well find that as you begin exercising consistently, you lose the desire to smoke. You become more conscious of your health and your lungs' capacity for endurance. Research shows that exercise can decrease the need to light up, because the extra oxygen needed during exercise reduces your nicotine cravings.
- Exercise helps you get a good night's sleep. That was the greatest benefit I received when I began exercising again during my recovery program. I hadn't had a good night's sleep in years. After a week, tension was reduced, my body tingled with fatigue, and sleep came to me like a welcome friend.
- Exercise helps you release tensions and alleviate stress. The side effects of stress, such as depression, anxiety, and fatigue, decrease.
- Sports psychology researchers have found that 20 to 30 minutes of aerobic exercise act as a "quick-fix" mood elevator. There is evidence that the body's natural opiates (beta-endorphins) are produced with a consistent exercise program. These chemicals increase tolerance for pain, decrease stress and anxiety, and produce a sense of euphoria.

Others claim that another hormone, noradrenaline, is present in higher concentrations during exercise and may elevate a person's mood.

EXERCISE ADDICTS

Exercise has such significant benefits that we who are accustomed to behaving in compulsive, addictive ways can actually become addicted to exercise. We have to learn not to O.D. on our fitness programs, thus abusing our bodies all over again.

There are definite signals that warn you that you are becoming an exercise addict:

- You can't and won't quit exercising more than you need to.
- You neglect meetings, job, and family.
- You continue exercising when you are in pain or are injured.
- If a doctor prescribes rest, you change doctors.
- You become depressed and fatigued from exercising too much.

Remember that the "easy does it" motto also applies to this phase of your recovery.

YOUR EXERCISE LOG

The following chapters describe how to set realistic goals. You will learn to congratulate yourself for completing a workout instead of damning yourself for not exercising more.

Begin by completing a daily Exercise Log. (A form for this is on page 212.) Don't alter your exercise habits for the first week. This initial log will be your baseline. In a few weeks, you'll be amazed at how much more active you are. Pay close attention to your emotions before and after you exercise. The typical workout might begin with feelings of boredom, tension, and fatigue, which lift as you begin moving aerobically. When you finish, you will feel energized, serene, and joyful (at least some of the time).

The following excerpts are from a letter from one of my clients, attesting to the benefits he has derived from exercise: "My name is Phil. I am an alcoholic. I am also a long-distance runner. I don't seem to be able to drink and run at the same time; whenever I have tried to do both, the drinking has prevailed.

"I ran track in high school and college until my running was terminated by tendonitis in my left knee. I started drinking when I was 20—mostly beer—and soon became an alcoholic, although I didn't discover that fact until much later. I was totally out of shape at 35, when my doctor ordered me to exercise—either jogging or handball. I chose jogging, and I discovered that I could do a mile if I mostly walked. I then weighed 234 pounds.

"Just before I turned 36, I quit drinking for the first time, because I thought I might be an alcoholic. When I was 36, I decided to become a Christian after 20 years of atheism, and I quit smoking for good just before I turned 37. My weight, which had gotten down to about 180, ballooned up to 210 when I substituted ice cream for cigarettes, but soon I got down to 170. During those two good years while I was jogging, I also changed jobs for the better and found a new woman.

"After the woman moved out, I said, 'To hell with it,' and quit jogging. Soon I was drinking heavily again. I was 38.

"When I was 41, I joined a therapy group. The therapist asked me to list three goals, no matter how wildly unobtainable. I wrote, 'Get married, run a marathon, and win a world bridge championship.' She said, 'I think you can do all of those things.' I then weighed 280 pounds, and I became obsessed with the marathon. I quit drinking in accordance with the therapist's orders.

"Within eight months, I lost 100 pounds, ran the Mission Bay Marathon, and was living with a new woman. My therapist was urging me to join A.A., but I didn't think I needed to. At the Natural Lite Half-Marathon, it was 100 degrees, and they had free beer. I decided one beer couldn't hurt me when I was so hot, so I had one. Within two weeks, I was drinking heavily again. The woman moved out, and I quit running.

"Anyway, I joined A.A. in 1980, and I had my last drink on

July 7, 1981, when I was 43, after a nine-day relapse which almost killed me. I don't drink, I go to A.A. meetings, and I run daily. My disease is mental, physical, and spiritual. For my physical recovery, I run and abstain from all drugs and sugar. Since June 1983, I have eaten only nutritious natural food, with the exception of cake from my wedding a week ago.

"My running helps with the other aspects of my recovery. When I run daily, I don't get depressed, and I used to get depressed a *lot*. Running is also when I do my meditation. I believe that the 12 steps of A.A. and my relationship with God are the keys to my recovery, but running and diet are essential, too."

ASSIGNMENTS

1. Complete your Exercise Log for one week, without changing your normal habits. If you aren't accustomed to exercising regularly, list the times you are most active during the day. Walking to work, climbing the stairs at home, or playing a game with friends are all physical activities that increase your fitness level.

2. Update your log as you initiate and follow through with your fitness program.

10
Your Self-Evaluation

*T*he fourth step in the 12-step recovery program of A.A. is to take a thorough moral inventory of oneself. We must do this to discard the self-defeating behaviors of our lives. We slowly start to substitute right living for wrong living. This step is at the very core of our recovery.

If you really want to get back into top physical condition, you must do something similar to the fourth step with your RRP Program. You can do this by evaluating yourself, by filling out all the charts and worksheets included in your program, and by reviewing them frequently.

YOUR RRP PROGRAM SELF-EVALUATION

First, be sure you have compiled all your questionnaires, worksheets, and logs in your RRP Program notebook. Thus far, your notebook should include the following:

- Your Self-Portraits
- Measurement Chart

- Daily Diet Diary
- Vitamin and Mineral Lists
- Exercise Log

When you finish this chapter, you will add the following to your RRP notebook:

- Your Health Evaluation—A review of your history of addiction and current health condition. Bring this with you when you visit your doctor for a complete physical.
- Your Physician's Checklist—A list of the basic health information you need in order to succeed with your RRP Program. Make an appointment with your doctor for a complete physical, and take this list along. As your doctor examines you, fill in the blanks on your form.
- Your Lifestyle Inventory—By answering these questions, you can learn how to integrate your fitness program into your lifestyle.
- Your Daily Inventory—This list gives you a daily measure of your success. Use it as a daily diary to complete before you go to bed. As you progress, compare your answers with those from the first days of your program. You will see how your lifestyle and attitudes are changing.
- Your Written Commitment—This is your promise to yourself to follow your RRP Program.

These forms are found in Appendix A, pages 213–21.

THE POWER OF PLANNING YOUR PROGRAM

By taking time out to complete your RRP Program notebook and self-evaluation, you enable yourself to formulate strategies to give you positive results. You become aware of the patterns of behavior that have been self-destructive. Your RRP Program notebook increases your commitment to health.

This phase of recovery is crucial to avoiding relapses. By evaluating yourself and your life in various ways, you learn about your many valuable qualities. When you make mistakes and procrastinate in the program, you become aware of your weaknesses, and strive to make those your strengths.

My clients find it helpful to write their programs on paper and chart their successes and goals. When they see their lives on paper, their whole program becomes more concrete to them. It gives them a point of reference for any changes needed to further their progress. By writing your plan down, you are giving yourself another gift in sobriety—a direction for your life.

When you make that written commitment to regain your health and keep it, you have taken one of the most important steps in your recovery. You have started to learn how to accept responsibility for administering your own health care program. You will experience, for the first time in years, a sense of self-control and discipline so important in your recovery.

Each day you participate in your program, you are actively deciding to become stronger mentally and physically. You will get to know your body, its likes and dislikes. You will accomplish things you never thought possible. When you experience the joys of fitness, you will wonder the same thing I did: Why in the world did I abuse my body when I could feel this good?

Regaining your health begins with one choice. You will either get into action or give up and die of your addiction. At this point, your success will be a matter of making intelligent choices and increasing your options.

Action, so often discussed in the Big Book of A.A., is the key to regaining your health. You need to keep logs and plan your new health care program in advance to eliminate the temptation to drink or use drugs to cope with the stress and emotional highs and lows of sobriety. If you don't have this plan worked out and the time comes when you get depressed, hungry, angry, lonely, and tired (H.A.L.T.), you will enter the danger zone in your recovery and could be setting yourself up for a slip. At times, troubles will drive you to the edge and push your stress level to a point of exploding, that point where you are no longer rational. When these situations present themselves, your *planned* program will help prevent you from heading toward that deadly drug or drink.

Above all, you must get rid of perfectionism and the need for instant success. Be patient with yourself as you go through these changes. Keep in mind the slogan "one day at a time" when you chart your program. Remember that the many hours you used up by drinking and using drugs need to be replaced with new and pleasurable experiences. Your whole body is trying to adjust.

You are learning to live in the now and to have fun all over again—without drugs and booze. You must not sit and think about what you are going to do. Take action. Follow this step-by-step plan, and you will truly find joy in sobriety.

ASSIGNMENTS

1. Review your RRP Program notebook. Be sure you have included all your lists, worksheets, and logs from the previous chapters.
2. Complete your Health Evaluation.
3. Make an appointment with your doctor. Bring your Health Evaluation and Physician's Checklist. Explain that you are learning about your health, and would like the doctor's evaluation of your condition. After your physician has completed the checklist, go over it and your other forms. Discuss your physical condition. Together, decide what changes you need to make.

11
Your Fitness Test

*W*hen I was writing this book, people often asked me, "What makes your book different from the many other fitness books on the stands?"

It is different because it is written by an alcoholic for other alcoholics and addicts. I have been a health and physical education teacher for most of my adult life and am able to teach subjects relevant to this disease. You might say that, when combined, these experiences have prepared me to present this program to those still suffering.

Alcoholics are different. Because of our addictions, we were spiritually, mentally, and physically sick. We are recovering from a devastating illness; our bodies have taken a tremendous beating. We are not just "normal" sedentary people who need to eat right and exercise regularly to gain our optimum level of fitness and health. We are starting at a much lower point; we have much damage to undo. We need a special approach to fitness and health, as outlined in this Recovery/Relapse-Prevention Program.

Our specialness does not, and must not, keep us from working as hard as we can to be as fit as we can be. It does not take tremendous insight to know that you are in terrible shape when you first begin your recovery. But to what extent have alcohol and drugs damaged your body? How fit are *you*? Do you really *know* what kind of shape you are in? How does your fitness level stack up against the rest of the population? Is it safe for you to exercise? To find the answers to these questions, take the tests in this chapter, by yourself or with the help of a recovering friend, and record your scores on the Personal Fitness Profile in Appendix A (page 222). Your scores will highlight your strengths and weaknesses, giving you a blueprint for your fitness program and goals.

Don't be surprised if your initial scores are lower than the median scores for "normal" test takers. It does not mean you cannot be healthy and fit. Every 30 days you will test yourself again and record your scores alongside those from your first tests. The differences may amaze you.

If you are in doubt about your health, check with a medical doctor before starting your testing or exercise program. Consult a doctor who understands the disease of addiction and the benefits of exercise. You will get more understanding and help.

YOUR CARDIOVASCULAR FITNESS TEST

Most of my clients are concerned about how long and how frequently they should exercise. Having heard a few too many stories about people who drop dead while they are exercising, they worry about straining their hearts. It is a valid concern, and one that can and should be considered frequently.

Everyone's cardiovascular capacity is unique. The answers to your exercise questions lie in your heart's capacity to meet the demands placed upon it. To determine how your heart is functioning, you must learn how to take your pulse. This simple procedure will help you gauge your heart rate, while resting and exercising. By interpreting your heart rate, you will know your heart's capacity.

To find your pulse, place three fingers lightly over the artery near the inside center of your wrist. Move your fingertips around until you feel the pulse. If you have trouble locating your pulse in your wrist, place two or three fingers along your neck about one inch below your jawbone. Using a stopwatch or the second hand on a wristwatch or clock, count the number of pulses for 15 seconds. Multiply this number by four to get your heart rate in beats per minute.

Test 1: Resting Heart Rate. The first measurement you need is your resting heart rate. The best time to take it is when you wake up in the morning. If your resting heart rate is over 100 beats a minute, consult your doctor immediately. Write your resting heart rate on your self-evaluation testing form, the Personal Fitness Profile.

RESTING HEART RATE

	Age			
	20–29	*30–39*	*40–49*	*50+*
Men				
Excellent	59 or less	63 or less	65 or less	67 or less
Good	60–69	64–71	66–73	68–75
Fair	70–85	72–85	74–89	76–89
Poor	86+	86+	90+	90+
Women				
Excellent	71 or less	71 or less	73 or less	75 or less
Good	72–77	72–79	75–79	77–83
Fair	78–95	80–97	80–98	84–102
Poor	96+	98+	99+	103+

Test 2: Step Test. The second test measures your maximum heart rate during exercise and your recovery heart rate after exercise. Together, they determine your aerobic fitness and stamina. This test reveals how fast your heart and lungs deliver oxygen to your body and how long it takes your pulse to slow down after it has

speeded up for exercise. This tells you how strong your heart is and helps you determine the effectiveness of your 30-day shape-up program. The sooner your heart returns to its resting rate, the better your condition. Make sure to write these scores on your self-evaluation testing form.

Step on a stair or stool about 8 inches high, then step down again, moving one foot after the other. Repeat 24 times a minute for three minutes. Stop and take your pulse. This gives you your maximum heart rate. If it is higher than those listed on the chart, consult a doctor before exercising aerobically.

After resting for 30 seconds, take your pulse again and consult the chart. Remember that as you get older, your heart's natural capacity will decline. If you feel dizzy, nauseous, or painfully breathless, stop!

SAFE MAXIMUM HEART RATE

	Age			
	20–29	*30–39*	*40–49*	*50+*
Men	170	160	150	140
Women	170	160	150	140

RECOVERY HEART RATE AT 30 SECONDS

	Age			
	20–29	*30–39*	*40–49*	*50+*
Men				
Excellent	74	78	80	83
Good	76–84	80–86	82–88	84–90
Fair	86–100	88–100	90–104	92–104
Poor	102+	102+	106+	106+
Women				
Excellent	86	86	88	90
Good	88–92	88–94	90–94	92–98
Fair	99–110	95–112	96–114	100–116
Poor	112+	114+	104+	118+

YOUR BODY FAT TEST

To be as fit as you can be, it is important to be the correct weight for your height. If you are overweight and lack flexibility, you can't be very mobile, and your weight will decrease your cardiovascular fitness. Besides, we know that obesity is associated with heart problems, diabetes, gall bladder diseases, and various types of cancer. Refer to the Standard Weight Table in Chapter 6 to determine what you should weigh.

Test 3: Measuring Your Body Fat. There are various elaborate tests to measure your body composition to determine how much fat you are carrying. Fat can be measured with calipers or underwater scales, but it really doesn't take that scientific an approach to decide if you are carrying too much fat. The pinch test described here works very well. As you exercise, the amount of fat you can feel on your body will diminish tremendously.

Pinch yourself at the waist and upper arm. Try to grab as much flesh as you can between your thumb and finger. If you can grab more than an inch, you will need to lose body fat.

YOUR FLEXIBILITY TEST

Strength and flexibility are two important ingredients to achieving all-around fitness. I will never forget all those moans and groans from the women I first worked with in the recovery house as they began their aerobic walking program. When we drank and "used," we were living sedentary lives. The next test will enable you to judge just how much your muscles, ligaments, and tendons have suffered from lack of use.

Test 4: Measuring Your Flexibility. Mark a starting line on the floor. Sit on the floor with your legs outstretched, your feet about six inches apart and your heels touching the line. Place a yardstick between your legs, perpendicular to the starting line, with the 15-inch mark at the line. Keep your heels on the line and your legs straight. With your hands stretched in front of you, slowly bend forward without straining or bouncing and touch the yardstick.

Note the measurement on the yardstick. Measure the space between your starting line (15 on the yardstick) and where your fingertips reached the yardstick. Score a plus figure if you are able to touch behind the heel, and a minus figure if you are not able to reach that far.

FLEXIBILITY

Men

	Age					
	Up to 35		36–45		46+	
Stretch Rating	cm.	in.	cm.	in.	cm.	in.
Excellent	+6	1½	+5	2	+4	1½
Good	−3	1¼	+2	¾	+1	1½
Fair	−5	2	−5	2	−6	2½
Poor	−8	3¼	−10	4	−10	4

Women

	Age					
	Up to 35		36–45		46+	
Stretch Rating	cm.	in.	cm.	in.	cm.	in.
Excellent	+8	3¼	+7	2¾	+6	2½
Good	+5	2	+4	1½	+3	1¼
Fair	−1	½	−3	1¼	−2	¾
Poor	−4	1½	−5	2	−6	2½

YOUR ENDURANCE AND STRENGTH TESTS

Endurance is a basic element of physical fitness. To maintain aerobic fitness, you need to sustain muscular effort without fatigue. Strength is necessary for you to healthfully participate in some form of recreational sport. Your goal is to determine whether your existing strength and muscular endurance are adequate to keep up with everyday living and leisure activities. In later chapters, you will find suggestions for developing and maintaining strength and muscular endurance.

Test 5: Sit-up Test. Lie on your back with your ankles firmly planted beneath a solid object or held by another person. Put your arms behind your head, and *with knees bent*, pull yourself up to a sitting position, using the strength of your stomach muscles. See how many sit-ups you can manage within 60 seconds, and consult the chart on page 86 to measure your result.

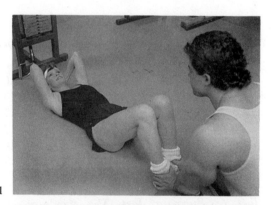

PHOTO 11-1

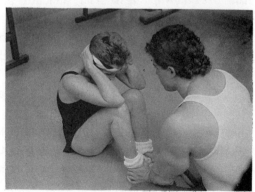

PHOTO 11-2

MUSCULAR ENDURANCE

Men

	Endurance Rating		
Age	*Excellent*	*Good*	*Poor*
12–14	45	35	25
15–19	50	40	30
20–29	40	30	20
30–39	35	25	20
40–49	30	20	15
50–59	25	15	10
60–69	23	13	8

Women

	Endurance Rating		
Age	*Excellent*	*Good*	*Poor*
12–14	44	34	24
15–19	40	30	20
20–29	33	23	13
30–39	27	17	12
40–49	22	12	7
50–59	20	10	5
60–69	17	7	4

Test 6: Push-up Test. The standard push-up test helps to determine your upper-body strength. Men usually do very well with push-ups, while many women lack the strength in their upper bodies to repeatedly perform them. Nevertheless, this test can help determine your overall body strength.

The push-up for men (see photos 11-3 and 11-4): Start in a front-leaning rest position, supporting your body on your hands and toes. Lower your body by bending at the elbows until your chest touches the floor. Keep your body flat and rigid. Return to the starting position. Your score is the number of correct, *complete* push-ups you can do.

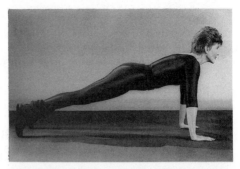

PHOTO 11-3

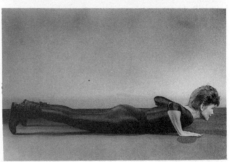

PHOTO 11-4

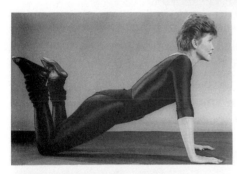

PHOTO 11-5

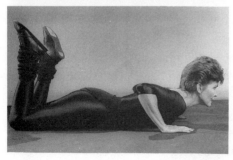

PHOTO 11-6

The push-up for women (see photos 11-5 and 11-6): Start in the depicted position and follow the instructions for the men's push-up. Don't worry if your score is low. You can include strength exercises for this area of your body when you set up your personal fitness program.

MUSCULAR STRENGTH AND ENDURANCE STANDARDS FOR ADULT MEN AND WOMEN

	Sit-Ups (60 Seconds)	Push-Ups (Front-Leaning Position)
Excellent	30 or more	15 or more
Good	25–29	10–14
Fair	20–24	5–9
Poor	Fewer than 20	Fewer than 4

THE NECESSARY INFORMATION

The self-evaluation tests suggested in this chapter are easy to do and can be successfully used for determining your fitness. Be sure to go through these tests carefully and accurately. Just as it is important in A.A. to be "thoroughly honest in all your affairs," so it is in this phase of your recovery. It is necessary to perform these tests correctly and record your true scores.

Now that you know what level you are at, you have the necessary information and motivation to set up your very own fitness program.

Don't forget to reevaluate your fitness level every 30 days, and to keep your personal fitness profile record current. Be sure to set realistic goals and remember: Progress, not perfection.

If you are over 35, you should have a medical evaluation incorporating a 12-lead electrocardiogram and blood pressure test. A blood profile and body composition test are additional helpful measures. You should have at least a five-hour blood glucose–tolerance test and liver enzyme test.

Please remember that "easy does it." Don't try to do too much too soon. If you completed this chapter precisely as it was laid out, you are on your way to carrying out a safe and beneficial fitness program. Use the charts provided to keep track of your training program.

ASSIGNMENTS

1. Complete your fitness tests. Fill in the Personal Fitness Profile (in Appendix A).

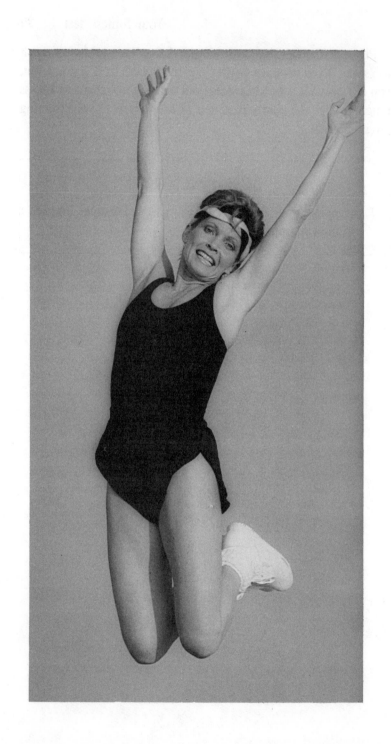

12
Your Aerobic Fitness Foundation

O nce you have completed your self-evaluation and fitness tests and have received approval from your doctor, you are ready to start exercising. By the time you finish this chapter, you will be walking and jogging regularly, and will be ready to start weight training and recreational sports.

Before you pull on your sweats and lace up your shoes, you must prepare your mind for the challenge ahead. You might be asking yourself some of the following questions. The answers will ensure confidence and success.

WHEN IS THE BEST TIME TO WORK OUT?

The best time to exercise is when you have time and can be sure to set aside a full hour for your workout.

Morning exercise gives the following benefits:

- You will have cleared your mind for the day's pressures and pleasures.

91

- You will begin your day feeling like you have succeeded at completing a worthwhile task. This feeling will carry through the day and result in improved performance and a sense of self-esteem.

Afternoon exercise gives the following benefits:

- You will clear the stress and anxiety that have built up in the morning.
- You will find others to join in your exercise. Some corporations have fitness lunch breaks to encourage employee well-being, because they know the payoffs are worth the investment. A fit employee is more productive, requires less sick leave, and has a positive mental attitude.

If you prefer to work out in the evening, be sure your exercise schedule does not conflict with your A.A. meetings. The benefits from evening workouts include:

- The chance to rid yourself of the stress, anxiety, anger, and frustration that may have built up during the day.
- The option of choosing a health club over a bar for unwinding after a hard day.
- Many people substitute eating for drinking as a stress reliever. When you exercise in the evening, you avoid the opportunity to soothe your feelings with food. Instead of stuffing your feelings, you drain off the negativity and enjoy the rewards of positive behavior.

WHERE SHOULD I WORK OUT?

When you are a beginner, the best place to start working out is in your home. By following the beginner's program in this book, you will slowly start to get in shape by walking or jogging in your neighborhood or at a nearby park or school track.

You can even set up your own home gym in your basement, den, or extra space. Home exercise equipment has become popular and is available at many price levels and in many styles.

Later, when your body needs more of a challenge and you are feeling more confident about your abilities, you can join a health club, exercise class, or YMCA/YWCA. Such places offer a variety of exercise options to keep your interest stimulated and your body challenged.

WHAT SHOULD I WEAR?

Exercise clothing is simple and inexpensive. The most important item is your shoes. Make sure they are well padded and comfortable, providing support without constricting movement. Test the shoe for flexibility. If it doesn't bend and stretch with your foot, don't wear it.

Good running shoes cost $20 to $60 and are worth the investment, but if you can't afford them at first, use standard sneakers or tennis shoes. Your initial workout will involve more walking than running, with less stress on your feet and legs. Still, once you start running, you need the support and comfort of a good running shoe. Poor shoes lead to poor performance and pain, which destroy the pleasurable benefits of exercise.

Some people prefer to run without socks, but if you run on pavement on a hot day, you'll soon find that your feet feel like they're on fire. It's OK to skip the socks if you're running on the beach or a soft surface, but use the extra padding of wool or cotton socks otherwise.

In warm weather, nylon shorts are cool and allow your skin to breathe. In the winter, switch to cotton for warmth. When it's really cold, wear sweat pants and sweatshirts that are loose and comfortable, without binding the ankles or waist.

When using equipment at a health club, wear clothing that covers your back and legs. No one likes to use a machine that's wet from someone else's perspiration. Many women prefer leotards and tights that allow for a wide range of movement. No matter what you wear, the most important considerations are comfort and freedom of movement.

HOW DO I AVOID MUSCLE SORENESS?

You won't get sore if you start your program slowly. Follow the warm-up exercises carefully, allowing your muscles to stretch and come alive, ready for harder work without pain.

If you experience severe pain, stop. Pain is the body's way of telling you that you are pushing too hard too fast. Relax the muscle and let it rest while exercising the rest of your body. Remember, pain means your body has been abused. Be kind and nurse it back to health slowly.

HOW OFTEN SHOULD I WORK OUT?

When you start your training program, you will be working muscles that have been inactive for a long time. They need to rest at least 24 hours after each workout. I recommend three times per week at first, with a full day off in between each session. After two or three months, you can boost your workout schedule to four days per week, using a combination of days that fits your personal schedule and alternates exercise and resting days.

WILL I DEVELOP BIG MUSCLES WORKING WITH WEIGHTS?

Every woman I have worked with has asked this question. The answer is no. To get big muscles, you would have to train at least four hours per day with heavy weights. Women have an extra layer of fat that keeps them from looking overly muscular. What you get from weight training is a beautiful body—fit and toned. The quickest and most satisfying results come from a program that combines aerobics, conditioning, and weight training.

WILL MY MUSCLES TURN TO FAT IF I STOP WORKING OUT WITH WEIGHTS?

Muscle tissue cannot be turned into body fat. That is impossible. But if you stop lifting weights, you must decrease your caloric intake. The less energy you expend and the more calories you consume, the fatter you will be.

WHAT IS AEROBIC EXERCISE?

Aerobic exercise is exercise that keeps your heart pumping near its maximum capacity for an extended period of time. Exercises that are aerobic are those that use the large muscle groups in your arms and legs continuously, without stopping. Walking, running, biking, and swimming are aerobic; they give you aerobic benefits when they are performed without stopping for 20 minutes. In these activities your cardiorespiratory system transports blood and oxygen to your muscles while removing lactic acid and carbon dioxide.

There is much discussion over how long and hard you have to work out to be getting aerobic benefits. The best gauge is to warm up, then move aerobically, with your heart beating fast but not so hard that you cannot carry on a normal conversation, and continue moving for over 20 minutes. Always cool down with stretches afterward.

Anaerobic exercise is that which is performed in bursts, rather than continuously. Weight lifting, sprinting, and sports such as tennis and racquetball get your heart pounding hard but provide breaks every few minutes, which allow your heart to slow down. Since they do not keep the heart rate up for an extended period of time, they are anaerobic.

YOUR AEROBIC WALKING PROGRAM

Now that you have the right clothing and have set up your exercise time, you are ready to begin your Aerobic Walking Program. You will learn basic warm-up and cool-down exercises and the fundamentals for your walking program. Some basic guidelines are:

- *Put some rhythm in your walk.* A good portable radio with a headset helps you keep walking at a steady pace. Swing your arms and lengthen your stride, keeping a rhythmic pace.
- *Keep a daily log.* Jot down the distance covered and the total time you walked.
- *Be aware of opportunities to walk.* Park far away from your office or home. Use stairs instead of elevators. During your lunch hour, eat for a half-hour and walk for a half-hour. Walk after dinner. Start programming yourself to increase your activity level daily.
- *Take steps to stop smoking and stick to your nutritional program.*

Warm-up Exercises. OK, let's go! You can warm up inside or outside. Be sure to do these exercises before you begin walking and again when you finish.

- *Toe touches*—Compare your position to that in photo 12-1. *Stretch very slowly*, reaching your arms high into the sky, then

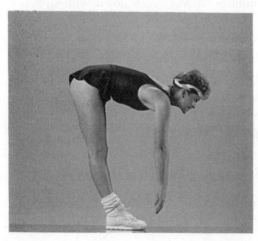

PHOTO 12-1

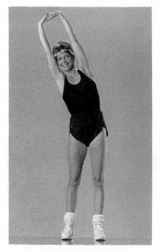 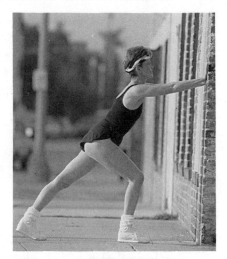

PHOTO 12-2   PHOTO 12-3

bending slowly from the waist toward the ground. Keep your knees straight, your heels flat on the floor. Don't worry if your fingers barely reach past your knees. Those muscles haven't been stretched for a long time. Stay relaxed, let your arms hang toward your feet, then stretch back up slowly, reaching toward the sky. Repeat five times.

• *Side bends*—Check photo 12-2. Stretch both arms into the air and interlace your fingers, palms facing the ceiling. Stretch to the right from the waist, keeping your torso facing forward. Stretch upright, then to the left. Repeat five times for each side.

• *Wall stretches*—Check photo 12-3. Place your palms against the wall, arms straight. Stretch your left arm back, keeping it straight while bending your right leg. Push your body away from the wall. Hold the stretch, then relax. Repeat five times. Switch legs and repeat stretch five times.

• *Hamstring stretches*—Check photo 12-4. Sit on the floor with your legs together in front of you, feet flexed and knees slightly bent. Stretch both arms straight over your legs as far as they will reach. Then roll back up slowly until you are sitting erect again. Repeat five times.

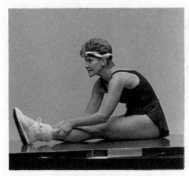

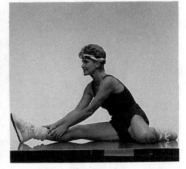

PHOTO 12-4   PHOTO 12-5

- *Hurdle stretches*—Check photo 12-5. This helps stretch the muscles in the lower back, hips, and thighs. Extend your right leg forward. Bend your left leg and place on the floor at the side of the hip. Lean forward over the straight leg, grabbing as close to the ankle as possible. Hold the stretch, then come back to sitting position. Repeat five times. Then change sides and repeat the stretch five times.
- *The turtle*—Check photo 12-6. This is good for the inner thighs, lower back, hamstrings, and buttocks. Starting position: Bend your legs and place your soles together, grasping your feet. Touch your chin to your chest and bend your body

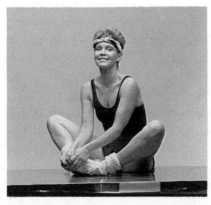

PHOTO 12-6

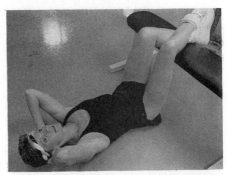

PHOTO 12-7

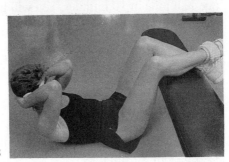

PHOTO 12-8

forward as far as it will go. While in this position, raise your head slowly. Come back to starting position, slowly arching your back.

• *The crunch*—Check photos 12-7 and 12-8. This is a good exercise for the muscles in front of the stomach. Lie on your back with your legs on top of a bench or chair. Place your hands behind your head. Slowly lift your back about eight inches off the floor. Hold for two seconds, then come back down slowly. Repeat five times.

Shake out your limbs, stretch a couple more times, and you're ready to walk.

At the end of every walk, repeat your warm-up exercises to help stretch fatigued and tight muscles. Proper warm-up and cool-down are essential to preventing injury and getting the most benefit from your workout.

THE SECRET: PROGRESS

The walk/run program is designed for slow progression. The secret is *progress*, not perfection. This is your exercise prescription for the next 30 days. Integrate your RRP Nutritional Program with your walking program, and you will start feeling a dramatic change in your life.

Week One. Once a day, three days per week, walk a distance of one-half mile in 10 minutes. You will be walking at a rate of about 3 miles per hour.

Week Two. Once a day, three days per week, walk a distance of 1 mile in 20 minutes.

Week Three. Once a day, three days per week, walk a distance of 1½ miles in 30 minutes.

By now you could be getting a little bored and probably want more of a challenge. It is time to start jogging. If you don't feel ready to run, continue increasing your walking mileage a half-mile every two weeks.

Week Four. Once a day, three days per week, jog one-quarter mile, walk one-half mile, jog one-quarter mile.

CONTINUING THE PROGRAM

Once you begin running, you will notice you have a distinct running style. To maximize your benefits, run with a heel-first action, pushing off the ball of your foot with each stride. Let your arms relax and curl your fingers into loose fists to help your running motion. Keep your body straight and relaxed. Start with short strides, lengthening as you progress. Breathe rhythmically— never hold your breath as you run.

Now that you are improving your physical condition and your cardiovascular and respiratory systems are functioning well, you are ready to increase your strength by adding weight training to your program. By completing the worksheets that accompany the next chapter, you will establish your personalized conditioning program, building strength, endurance, flexibility, and confidence.

ASSIGNMENTS

1. Begin your walking program and monitor your progress.

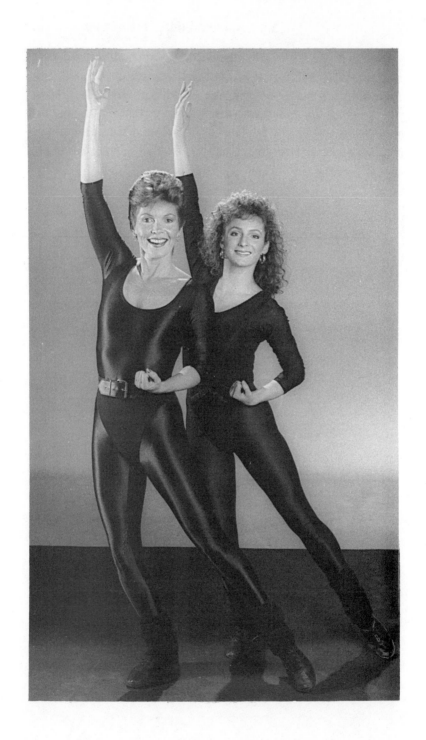

13
Your Physical
Fitness Foundation

*T*otal fitness includes aerobics, strength training, and sports. When you compile your Weekly Exercise Worksheet, you will include aerobics with a walking program, strength training with the exercises presented in this chapter, and sports and recreational activities from the next chapter. With a complete program, you will improve your cardiovascular fitness, strengthen and tone your body, and learn to enjoy being active.

When I returned to a regular fitness program, I felt my health being restored. I noticed the huge difference exercise was making in my life. My head cleared up, and I felt the veil of fog lifting slowly from my eyes. The world took on a special, sparkling clarity. I could think clearly, and I felt calm. The highs and lows disappeared. I had a tremendous amount of energy, which was refueled by my weight-training program. I started to feel strong and confident. My blotchy, alcoholic look was replaced with beautiful, glowing skin. I became more aware of the foods I should eat and became quite health-conscious. The people I work with experience the same results.

After a year of exercising regularly, I felt confident enough to compete in the weight-lifting event at the Alcoholic Olympics. I competed and won! This year (my fourth year), I competed outside of an alcoholic event and was runner-up in the over-40 women's weight-lifting and clean-jerk contest for the state of California. I was five years older than the winner, and I have truly never felt more fit in my whole life.

Self-respect and fitness go hand in hand. How can you create a beautiful, healthy body and be full of self-hate? You will learn something valuable through your new program—you will learn to *love* yourself! The clients I work with feel better when their bodies regain health and strength. They are no longer victims of their disease, but individuals with rights, in control. This is not fantasy, but fact. Physical fitness allows you to experience that you are, at last, doing something for yourself.

GUIDELINES FOR FITNESS

Guidelines for physical fitness have been outlined by the President's Council on Physical Fitness. The components covered are endurance, strength, and flexibility. Endurance enables you to use energy for a long period of time. Strength determines how much force a muscle can produce. Flexibility determines how much range of movement a joint can perform. These three basic principles augment your aerobic fitness. By following them, you learn how to exercise for maximum benefits.

Frequency. In the beginning, you should work out three days a week, with "rest" days in between each workout. You rest to give your body a chance to recover. It is important to exercise every other day, and not skip two or three days in a row. Your body maintains its fitness level for only a short period of time, then slips back to its former sedentary condition. If you allow too much time to elapse between workouts, you don't get to see and feel the results that come from a consistent program. You will not be able to achieve your fitness goals.

Intensity. During your workouts, your heart should be beating fast and hard to enhance your cardiovascular efficiency. The intensity of exercise is measured at 75 percent of your maximum heart rate (HR). The range for most adults is 100–120 HR beats a minute. Most adults can work out comfortably at this level of intensity, once they become fit. When your heart is beating hard, you will notice an increase in perspiration and more rapid breathing, though you should still be able to carry on a conversation at a normal level.

If you have an aerobic program with this intensity, you will get your desired results. If you exercise below this level, you will show little change in your cardiorespiratory fitness level. If you keep the intensity of your fitness program moderate, you will enjoy your activity more. At the same time, you will eliminate injury and find it easier to stick with your program.

Duration. The energy you expend is directly related to the duration of your exercise. The ideal duration time is 30 minutes of aerobic exercising in the beginning, eventually going to 60 minutes. You will soon recognize how the frequency and duration of your fitness program directly affect your fitness level.

Take a look at the energy level expended in running as opposed to walking. Although the energy cost for running is much higher than walking, the aerobic walking program outlined in this book can be as effective as running for improving your cardiorespiratory function. If you want your fitness level to progress and can exercise for only 15 minutes, you would require a high-intensity workout. If you have a longer time to work out, you can approach it in a more leisurely fashion.

STRETCHING

Stretching increases the flow of blood to your muscles and improves the range of motion around your joints. This increases your athletic performance and decreases your chances of injury.

Yoga is an excellent activity that uses quite a bit of stretching to increase your flexibility and promote meditation. Several yoga books and classes are available; whether or not you decide to include yoga in your fitness program, it is a good idea to learn about this discipline and incorporate its tenets of balance and harmony into your life. I recommend yoga highly. It incorporates relaxation and enlightenment through the control exerted over one's own body.

Stretching is an integral part of conditioning and should be used before and after your workouts. Stretching can also extend into a 20- to 30-minute time period—actually constituting a workout.

Hold your stretches ten seconds and repeat five times. Stretching should be done within your limits and should be enjoyable. Stretching is a graceful, gradual movement. Don't bounce or jerk your limbs into place. Instead, reach for the sky or the ground with a slow, even movement, allowing gravity to help you reach farther and farther. Breathe slowly and deeply as you stretch.

Here are some good basic stretches to start out with:

- *Toe touch, straight-legged*—See photo 13-1. Stand and slowly bend forward, slightly bending the knees. Allow your arms to dangle loosely. Hold for ten seconds. Keep head relaxed and back slightly rounded.

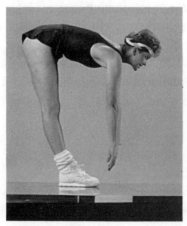 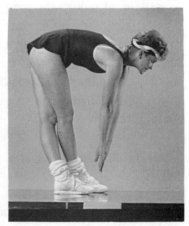

PHOTO 13-1   PHOTO 13-2

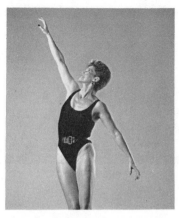

PHOTO 13-3

- *Toe touch, cross-legged*—See photo 13-2. Stand straight and cross your left foot over your right foot. Bend over and stretch your hands to the toes of your left foot. Hold for ten seconds. Stand up slowly and cross opposite feet. Repeat five times for each side.
- *Side stretch*—See photo 13-3. Stand with your feet together, knees slightly bent. Reach up with your right arm and down with your left arm. Look up toward your raised arm. Repeat on the other side, reaching up with your left arm and down with your right arm. Feel the stretch. Repeat five times for each side.
- *Hamstring stretch*—See photo 13-4. Sit on the floor with your legs together in front of you, feet flexed and knees slightly bent. Stretch both arms straight over your legs as far as they will reach. Don't hold your breath. Then roll back up slowly until you are sitting erect again. Repeat five times.
- *Hurdle stretch*—See photo 13-5. Sit on the floor. Stretch your left leg forward, and bend your right leg back at an angle. Stretch both arms out toward your left foot. Hold for ten seconds, stretching and lengthening your left side. Don't bounce. Switch legs and repeat five times for each side.
- *Groin stretch*—See photo 13-6. Sit on the floor with your knees apart and the soles of your feet together. Draw the feet back toward the groin. Grasp the feet at the instep or ankle

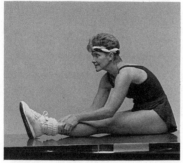

PHOTO 13-4

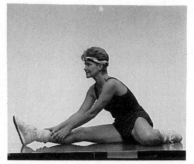

PHOTO 13-5

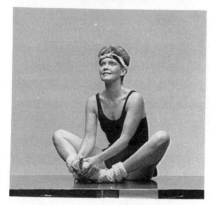

PHOTO 13-6

with both hands. Slowly lean forward, keeping your back flat and continuing to draw the feet back toward the groin. Hold stretch for ten seconds, then slowly come to upright position. Repeat five times.

WEIGHT TRAINING

When I first started regaining my health, the minute I entered a gym, my worries left. I discovered weight training—an activity that would profoundly affect the quality of my sobriety. I was 44 years old and shaped my body into one that brought the envy of 18-year-olds. I developed enough strength to enter competitions in weight lifting and win! I truly felt I retarded my aging process. I developed a sense of accomplishment and a certain kind of control over my life.

The following program is the one I excelled in and feel most evangelistic about. One of the best ways to regain your self-esteem and gain self-confidence is through weight training. It feels good; you feel strong, supple, vibrant, and in control. You develop a better understanding of your body, and you gain a subconscious desire not to abuse your body ever again. You will notice radical differences and changes in your body in comparison to how it used to feel during your drinking and drugging days.

I met other people who did not drink or use drugs. I made friendships that were nurturing. Everyone seemed to want to help each other become the very best they could be. I had found another kind of support group that cared about my progress. I regained all I had lost physically, mentally, and spiritually inside those gyms. My enthusiasm for weight training permeates the fitness programs I design for my clients. I promote health through weight training.

Weight training firms and tones the muscles, shaping the body. For weight training, there are two basic kinds of equipment: Universal and Nautilus machines and free weights. The exercises

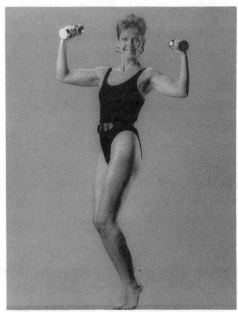

PHOTO 13-7

using each type of equipment are performed with a certain number of repetitions in each set. A set equals a number of repetitions performed in sequence, followed by a 40-second rest period.

Universal and Nautilus Machines. These pieces of equipment use adjustable stacks of weights. They feature constant resistance for a thorough workout throughout your entire range of motion.

To determine the amount of weight right for you, set the weights (usually in five-pound increments) to the point where you can comfortably perform five to ten repetitions.

Breathing techniques are essential. Exhale as you lift the weights, and inhale as you lower them. Never rest the weights on the stacks between repetitions; just let the weights touch the stack briefly before doing another rep. Never complete a repetition in less than two seconds. If you do, the weights will move at their own momentum, making the exercise less productive. When the reps get easy, add 10 pounds and another set if time permits.

Free Weights. The big difference between strength training with free weights versus machines is that you can exercise *specific* parts of the body. The range of movement is limited only by the body's range. You develop greater coordination, because you have to concentrate on controlling the direction of the weights.

YOUR WEIGHT-TRAINING ROUTINE

The basic information on weight training in this chapter forms the foundation for rebuilding your strength and reshaping your body. You will experience the best results if you follow the guidelines carefully.

Proper Form. To get the maximum benefit out of each exercise, use form that places maximum stress on your muscles. To accomplish this, follow the performance guidelines with each pictured position. For maximum results, use only the muscles that are supposed to be exercised, leaving the rest of the body motionless.

Move the barbell or weight *slowly* along the full range of motion allowed by the joints during the exercise.

Avoid using quick, jerky movements; raise and lower the weight slowly. If you tend to drop the weight, you will not benefit from the exercise.

Follow the pictures exactly, exercising in front of a mirror to check your position.

Beginner's Muscle Soreness. This program deliberately eliminates muscle soreness. If you do the warm-ups and cool-downs set forth in this program, you can eliminate the soreness that most beginners experience. If you limit your sets to two and keep your repetitions from eight to ten, chances are muscle soreness will be minimal.

If you start feeling sore, rest your muscles. Don't push yourself into pain. If muscle soreness persists, frequent warm baths are the best antidote. If the pain is serious or you think you have strained or sprained a muscle, do not apply heat. Get your injury checked by a doctor.

Lower-Body Exercises (Hips and Thighs). Lunges (see photo 13-8) are a great exercise for firming and strengthening the thighs, hips, and hamstrings.

- Hold a barbell behind your neck. Stand with your feet eight to ten inches apart, toes pointing straight ahead.
- Keeping your body straight, step forward about four feet with your right foot. With your left leg held straight, slowly bend your right leg as much as possible.
- At the bottom of the movement, your right knee should be several inches in front of your left ankle. You should feel a stretching in your thigh muscles.

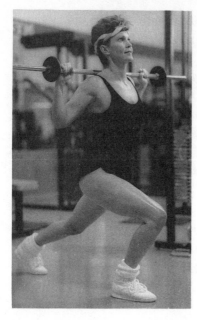

PHOTO 13-8

- Slowly straighten your right leg and push back to your starting position.
- Do your next repetition by stepping forward with the left foot. Alternate feet until you have completed the required number of repetitions.
- If the barbell is too awkward behind your neck, hold two light dumbbells down at your sides.

Leg extensions (see photos 13-9 and 13-10) work the quadriceps, the large muscles in the front of the thigh.

- Sit on the seat of the machine. Hook the front of your ankles under the set of roller pads.
- Straighten your legs until they are horizontal.
- Now lower your legs back to the starting position.

Leg curls (see photo 13-11) work the muscles in back of the legs. These muscles are called the biceps of your thighs.

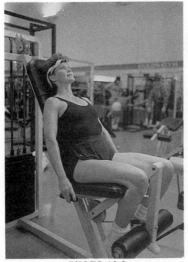

PHOTO 13-9

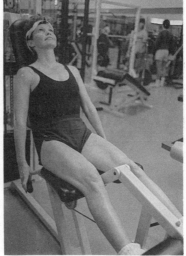

PHOTO 13-10

- Lie face down on the machine and slide your body down until your knees are on the edge of the pad. Hook your heels under the roller pads. Grab hold of handles provided for support.
- Curl your feet upward as fully as possible. Hold this for a second, and then *slowly* bring them back to a starting position.

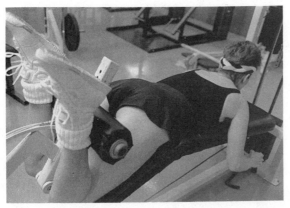

PHOTO 13-11

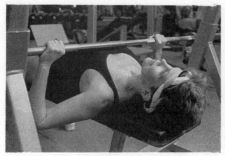

PHOTO 13-12

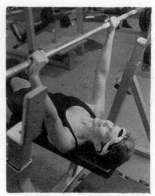

PHOTO 13-13

Chest. Bench presses (see photos 13-12 and 13-13) stress the pectorals, deltoids, and triceps.

- Place a barbell on the rack. Make sure you start out with the right weight, one you can easily press eight to ten times.
- Lie down on the bench, placing your feet flat on the floor. Grab the bar with your hands placed four or five inches farther apart than your shoulders.
- Straighten your arms to take the weight off the rack, and balance the barbell, bringing it to your chest, barely touching the breast bone.
- Press the barbell up again until your arms are locked out.

Shoulders. Military press (see photos 13-14 and 13-15): Place the barbell on the floor. Bend over, keeping your back flat. Grab the barbell with an overhand grip, with your hands set about six inches wider on each side than the width of your shoulders. Pull the barbell up to your chest, rotating your elbows under the bar. Don't let your body sway. Slowly push the barbell directly upward past your face, until your arms are locked out directly above your head. Slowly lower the barbell back to your starting point. Repeat until the required number of repetitions are completed.

Upright Rowing (see photo 13-16): Grab a barbell with a

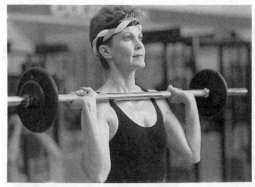

PHOTO 13-14

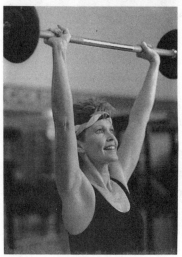

PHOTO 13-15

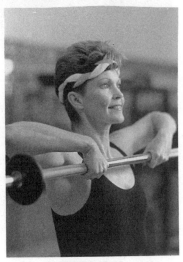

PHOTO 13-16

narrow overhand grip. Your thumbs should be about six inches apart. Stand straight and have your arms hanging down at your sides so the barbell and your hands rest across your upper thighs. From this starting position, slowly pull the bar upward, close to your body all the way up until it touches your chin. Be sure to keep your elbows high at the top of this movement. Slowly lower the barbell back to the starting point. Repeat the required number of times.

Back. *Back lat pull-downs* (see photos 13-17 and 13-18) are a

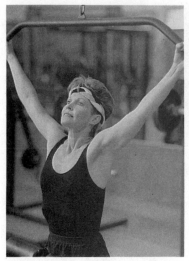
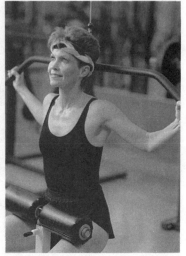

PHOTO 13-17   PHOTO 13-18

good exercise for the latissimus dorsi muscles and the upper back. Make sure your back stays straight as you do these.

- Place the pin in the appropriate weight.
- Next, grab the bar with palms facing away from the body, slightly farther apart than your shoulders. Hold the bar at arm's length above you, stretching your "lats."
- Pull the bar down behind your neck, barely touching the base of it.
- Let the bar *slowly* return to your starting position.

Arms. Barbell curls (see photo 13-19) work the biceps and some flexor muscles on the inner part of your forearms.

- Grab the barbell with an underhanded grip. Make sure your hands are about shoulder width apart, with upper arms pressed against the sides of your body. Keep them in this position throughout the whole exercise.
- Raise the bar out and up, curling it toward the chin.
- Slowly lower the bar until your arms are fully extended at your sides.

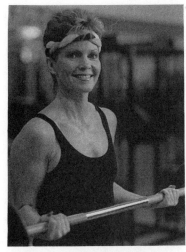

PHOTO 13-19

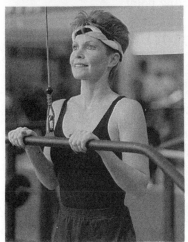

PHOTO 13-20

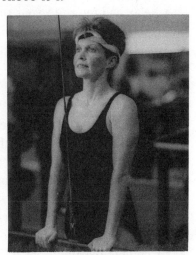

PHOTO 13-21

Pulley push-downs (see photos 13-20 and 13-21) are great for your triceps.

* Standing, grab the bar with an overhand grip. Place the hands a few inches apart. Keep your elbows at your sides.
* Slowly straighten your arms, keeping your elbows at your sides. Push the bar down until your arms are fully extended. Don't let your body sway. Keep it steady.

Stomach. Everyone I work with stresses the need for stomach exercises more than any other.

The crunch (see photo 13-22) is the first and best exercise to get your stomach muscles back into shape. This exercise affects the rectus abdominal muscles, particularly the upper abdominals ("abs").

* Lie on your back with your legs draped over a flat bench. Place your hands behind your head. Raise your shoulders from the bench, using your upper abs.
* Force your shoulders forward and exhale, contracting your abs at the top of the movement. Be sure to contract, rather than expand, your abdomen.
* Relax and return to your starting point.

Twists with a stick (see photos 13-23 and 13-24) are the greatest for getting rid of "love handles." This exercise helps loosen up the muscles in the lower back.

* Sit near the end of a flat exercise bench, feet flat on the floor. Hold a broomstick or light bar across the back of your shoulders. Wrap your arms around the top of it.
* Look *straight ahead* the entire time, and don't let your hips move. Twist your shoulders slowly as far as you can to the left. Then, without stopping, twist back as far as possible to the right.
* Continue twisting from side to side for about two minutes.

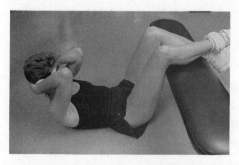

PHOTO 13-22

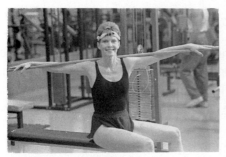

PHOTO 13-23

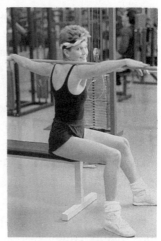

PHOTO 13-24

Sit-ups: Lie on your back, with your feet hooked under a piece of furniture, or have someone hold your feet steady. Bend your knees and lock your hands behind your neck. Keeping your elbows in, raise your body and bring your head as close to your knees as you can. Lower yourself back down and repeat.

YOUR PERSONAL WEIGHT-TRAINING PROGRAM

Before you start weight training, you will have to decide whether you want to work out in a club or in your home. Many of my clients lack the time to get to their health clubs regularly. Since I train many celebrities recovering from addiction and their desire for confidentiality is important, I do train them in their homes. There are still others who like home gyms as an alternative routine. They still go to their health clubs, but find that the variety keeps them from getting stale.

Before you go out and buy expensive equipment, you should consider the following questions:

• Are you planning on doing all your training at home? Do you plan to coordinate your home workouts with visits to your health club?

- Do you have the finances to purchase the latest state-of-the-art equipment? Have you familiarized yourself with the various price ranges of equipment?
- Do you have enough space to set up a home gym?
- Do you know how to use the equipment?
- Who will be using the equipment?

After you answer these questions, you will be in a position to make a decision about setting up a home gym. If you decide to supplement your regular sessions at your health club, then you can get by with a minimum amount of equipment. If you decide to set up your own gym and do all your training at home, you'll need to buy quality equipment.

One of the services I provide for my clients is assisting them in setting up their home gym. I suggest how easy it is to start out on a small budget. There are various resources such as the classifieds, recycler bargain papers, and swap meets.

If you are ready and willing to part with your dollars (consider it an investment in your health), you should browse around stores specializing in equipment for weight training. Check the salesperson's qualifications before you buy anything. Find out if the store employs people with backgrounds in physical education or exercise physiology. Does the salesperson work out with weights?

If you feel you need more direction and want to get the most knowledge available, hire a personal trainer. Try to get someone who knows about your disease from a health standpoint. Check credentials and make sure this person knows what he or she is doing. There are many professional body builders who subsidize their training by coaching others. I have found these people to have a vast storehouse of knowledge and to be excellent teachers. The average trainer charges $50 an hour. Think about it; it may be just what you need.

As you start this program, make sure that you perform every exercise precisely as you are instructed. Slowly increase the number of sets and pounds.

Most people I work with find they are able to add five to ten pounds, plus another set, within their thirty-day training program. Use the following workout for thirty days, three times a week.

Exercise	Sets	Reps
Crunches	1	10–20
Twisting	1	2 min.
Leg extensions	2	10–12
Leg curls	2	10–12
Flat bench press	2	8–10
Barbell shoulder press	2	6–8
Upright rows	2	6–8
Back lat pull-downs	2	8–10
Barbell curls	2	8–10
Pulley push-downs	2	8–10

YOUR WEIGHT-TRAINING DIARY

I found that I attained my best results by keeping a log of my workouts. I call this my training diary. The training diary is a valuable and revealing tool. Few people see changes in their fitness and strength levels on a day-to-day basis. With a training diary, you can easily see the effects of your training and nutritional program on your body. After practicing the various exercises listed, fill in the blanks on your Training Diary (on pages 224–25), developing your weight-training program. Add new exercises and increase your weights, sets, and reps as you grow stronger.

ASSIGNMENTS

1. Set up your exercise schedule.
2. Decide whether to assemble a home gym or join a health club.
3. Fill out your Training Diary, using your personal training program. Update your diary every week.

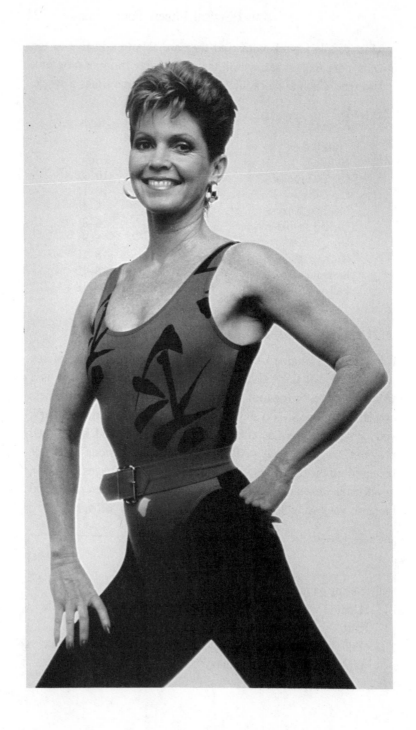

14
Exercise for Fun

Your physical recovery should be fun. The clients I work with who have the most success are the ones who find a special sport they enjoy. They use the sport as a form of self-expression and emotional release and are gratified by the results. They rarely get bored and look forward to their fitness program with excitement. I can tell you now that the most important factor in integrating fitness as part of your recovery is the sport or activity you choose to participate in regularly.

Believe it or not, most people I have worked with thought that exercise + sport = jogging. Few got very excited about that. They hadn't thought of all the other ways they could strengthen and tone their muscles and tune up their hearts and lungs. As we explored their preferences regarding exercise, they discovered activities they had enjoyed years ago that they could still be enjoying now.

Each sport has its benefits and drawbacks. Jogging is popular because it is inexpensive and less time-consuming than other activities. But so are many other forms of recreation—biking, walking, swimming, dancing. All of these activities are fun and

123

have countless physical rewards. The following descriptions enumerate the benefits of some of the more popular physical activities that can enhance your fitness and health.

WALKING

Walking is the best initial exercise for out-of-shape bodies. It helps build stamina and endurance, improves circulation, and helps get your legs in shape. Walking also helps reduce anxiety and tension and burns off body fat.

All of my clients begin with an aerobic walking program and find it easy to fit into their new daily living routines. I have outlined this aerobic walking program in Chapter 12. To obtain results, you should be consistent in using this program.

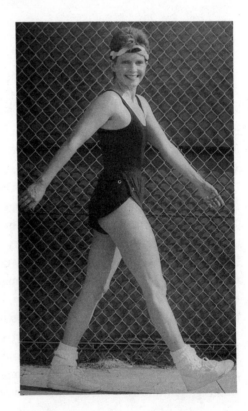

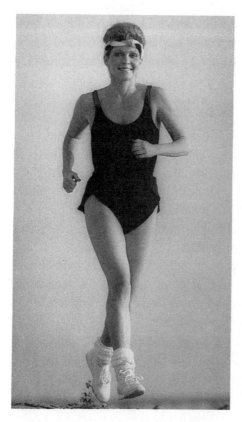

RUNNING AND JOGGING

Joggers notoriously have a minimal amount of body fat. Running
is one of the most intense aerobic workouts you can get. It is very
good for your cardiovascular conditioning and for developing the
lower body. You can run anywhere, anytime, with a few precautions for weather and safety. Just lace up your shoes and move on
out.

Many of my clients like the sense of freedom it gives them. They
enjoy having the opportunity to discover the different elements of
their neighborhoods that they were too "unconscious" to notice
before. They have a real sense of discovery and adventure that they
had not previously experienced.

If you have healthy knees, feet, and back, this is an ideal sport for you. However, most recovering alcoholics will need to follow the walking program in Chapter 12 before getting into a running program.

CYCLING

Almost everyone I work with eventually purchases a bike. In some parts of the country, they can take full advantage of extensive bike-path systems and year-round beautiful weather. The greatest rewards they experience as they gain confidence on their bikes is a tremendous sense of fun and childishness in its most positive sense. Fitness seems to be a fringe benefit.

Cycling is a rhythmic sport. It requires a sense of balance and timing that encourages a feeling of meditation. As your skills improve, you don't have to guide your body as it exercises. Once you catch on, you just bike automatically.

Like walking, bicycling is easy to fit into your schedule. I live about a mile from the health club where I work and ride my bike there every morning. Sometimes I get to work faster than my co-workers, who are stuck in traffic jams, and I certainly feel more invigorated and energized.

Physically, biking gives you great cardiovascular benefits and little danger of serious muscle or joint injury. It is a good sport for those who are overweight, since your ankles and knees are not directly bearing the brunt of your weight against concrete or asphalt. The only real dangers inherent in bike riding are those from accidents, which you can avoid if you abide by your local biking regulations and wear a helmet.

SWIMMING

Research repeatedly shows that swimming is one of the most popular recreational sports. I have taught swimming for years and must stress that for swimming to be a fitness sport, you must have

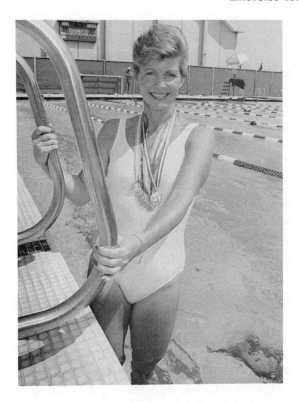

the proper swimming stroke and swim for at least a half-hour. When you are able to swim laps effortlessly for 30 minutes or more, you will start seeing the fitness benefits of swimming.

Most local YMCAs, YWCAs, and public pools have adult swimming classes for beginners and those who want to perfect their form. If you plan to use swimming for cardiovascular fitness, take one of these classes and learn how to get the most from each stroke.

The rhythmic, powerful movements and sensual pleasures of swimming quickly release your mind from the tedious details of life, and you will find yourself floating in a world of tranquility and relaxation, a state you thought you could reach only with alcohol and/or drugs. Yes, you can get high without using chemicals.

CROSS-COUNTRY SKIING

Cross-country skiing is a true total-body conditioner. It builds and tones the upper and lower body and has an extraordinary effect on your cardiovascular system.

Cross-country skiing is an endurance sport that basically consists of walking on skis. The hypnotic effect of the gliding is a mood enhancer and stress reducer. If you ski at a steady pace for an hour, you can burn 500 calories or more.

This is a seasonal sport and requires you to be in top condition. Consider cross-country skiing later on when your body can cope with intense physical demands. It is wonderful when you can strap on a pair of skis, glide out into nature, and enjoy the solitude and serenity without having to fight ski-lift lines.

AEROBIC DANCING

Aerobic dancing is popular with my clients, both male and female. Alone, it gives a good aerobic workout and helps strengthen the limbs. When combined with a weight-training program to tone and firm muscles, it gives a complete workout. In every city, there are programs at beginner, intermediate, and advanced levels.

It is important that aerobics classes begin with a warm-up period, stretching the muscles and allowing the heart rate to gradually climb to its maximum. The class should end with a cool-down to allow the heart to return gradually to its resting rate. Low-impact aerobics on padded floors helps decrease the chance of injury.

Aerobic dancing is a good activity for those who wish to exercise at home. Numerous cassettes and videotapes for you to follow are on the market. Be sure to use an exercise mat to decrease the impact, and follow the directions completely. It helps to watch yourself in a mirror to be sure your body is in the same position as the instructor's. And test your heart rate before, during, and after your workout.

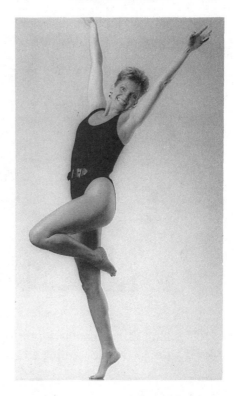

Aerobics classes are good for those in recovery. They offer a healthy atmosphere for socializing and provide a chance to dance without going to bars or clubs. They also meet the need for aerobic fitness. Best of all, they are fun.

Nonimpact and low-impact aerobics classes are the best for beginners, because they reduce the incidence of the injuries that prevail in more advanced regular aerobic classes. Nonimpact aerobics was recently instituted at the club where I work as a private trainer, and I recommend these classes to all my clients. Low-impact classes have the same format as regular aerobics classes, but discourage the jumping, jogging, and other jarring movements so prevalent in other aerobics classes. The nonimpact aerobics are done in place, and arm movements are combined with stepping to raise the heart rate. Low-impact and nonimpact

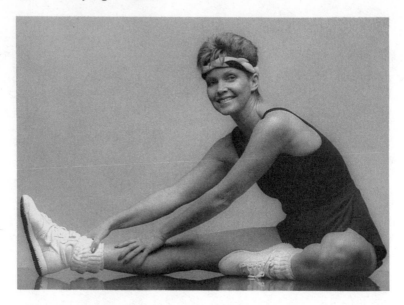

aerobics have gained popularity throughout the country, and you should have no trouble locating a class.

CALISTHENICS

Calisthenics are a form of strength training. They are especially helpful for beginners who want to start weight-training programs but haven't yet built up their strength. It is very important to perform calisthenic exercises properly to avoid injury and gain the most benefits.

Calisthenics are most familiar these days as exercises done to music. This form of rhythmic exercises can be seen in any aerobics class. Performed by themselves, calisthenics are not totally aerobic, but are useful for any strength-training program.

ROWING AND CANOEING

Rowing and canoeing are excellent forms of aerobic exercise. These require strength and energy. You should view them as alternatives as you progress. Rowing demands back strength and requires good techniques to avoid back injuries.

HIKING

Hiking is great for getting outdoors and enjoying nature. Through the sheer enjoyment this activity provides, you can face obstacles that will test your physical agility. Hiking has become an increasingly popular sport, and it is one I recommend highly.

TENNIS

I love tennis and am partial to this sport. I used to teach tennis at John Gardiner's Tennis Ranch in Carmel Valley. I have played this sport for many years and love the overall body conditioning it produces. Tennis is also a good way to increase your circle of health-oriented friends. You can play tennis anywhere in the world as long as you have decent weather.

GOLF

This is another favorite sport of mine. Golf is excellent for developing eye-hand coordination but lousy for conditioning. Sure, you walk a lot, but most people I know take golf carts. Still, I enjoy playing this game, particularly in beautiful surroundings.

A word of caution. Golf is time-consuming and fairly expensive. You could cut your costs by getting a city permit and playing at a public course. One of the advantages of playing this game is that you don't have to have a partner, you can play alone or become part of an existing group. If I don't take this game too seriously, I find it to be an excellent form of relaxation. I have also met some wonderful people on the many golf courses I have played on.

INTEGRATING SPORTS INTO YOUR RRP PROGRAM

Sports are but one aspect of your total fitness program. Most have cardiovascular and strengthening benefits. To maximize the benefits, particularly if you are interested in toning and shaping your body, you should combine your sport with a strength-training program such as weight lifting. You will then be able to achieve the maximum results to achieve your fitness goals.

You need to be in shape to enjoy the sport you choose. The longer you play, the greater the cardiorespiratory benefits. The more often you participate in the sport you enjoy the most, the faster you will improve your conditioning program.

To enjoy your sports activity and look forward to it as playtime, include it in your weekly schedule and treat it as you would any other important appointment. Schedule it in place of other workouts three or four times a week, in writing. If you don't, obstacles and other priorities will invariably arise to push aside your fitness program. Schedule your playtime and take charge of your health and lifestyle.

The activity you choose can literally change the quality of your sobriety. As your body, mind, and spirit develop and you begin to experience a balance in your life, you will experience the true meaning of a great A.A. slogan, "Happy, joyous, and free." Dennis K.'s testimony says it all:

"I was lucky. By remaining active throughout the course of my drinking, I warded off many of the physical effects of alcoholism. But there was a discernible and continuous drop in the quality of my performances, until one day I simply fell off my bicycle. My reflexes and coordination were going. This event made it clear that my general health was in danger. I could no longer count on athletics to buffer my drinking.

"The differences today are startling. I am capable of things today that 10 years ago, while drinking, I could not do. And the by-products of sports in sobriety have truly enhanced my life. I've acquired an outlet for unresolved emotions, a vehicle of 'being part of,' and I've learned how to play. I've achieved a sense of well-being, a balanced and appropriate self-esteem, and a newfound meaning of the word *fun*.

"The disease of alcoholism manifests itself in three ways: spiritually, emotionally, and physically. So the recovery has to address each of these, on equal terms. In my recovery, each leg of the triad feeds off the others and complements the others. If my recovery did *not* include sports, I would probably be sober, but I'd also probably be miserable."

ASSIGNMENTS

1. Practice playing actively. Try out the activities listed in this chapter, and choose a few that suit you best. Incorporate them into your weekly schedule.

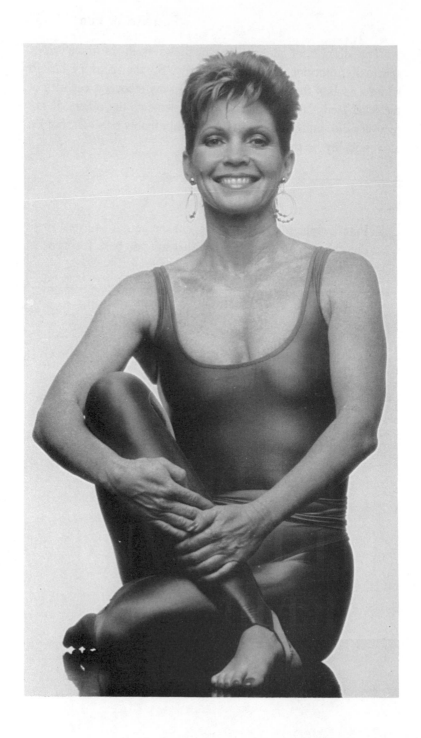

15
Your Self-Styled Fitness Program

As you begin to follow your conditioning and aerobic fitness programs, you will quickly feel the results. Your renewed health and vitality will motivate you to continue following and updating your personal fitness program, geared to your interests. age. and fitness level.

YOUR FITNESS FOUNDATION

In the previous chapters, you learned about aerobics, strength training, and sports and recreation. Now it is time to combine all three in your total RRP Fitness Program.

In Appendix A is your Weekly Exercise Worksheet (page 223), with blank lines for you to fill in your exercise plans. To completely tone your body, improve your health, and protect yourself from injuries, you need to include exercise under all categories.

• Stretching—Consult Chapters 12 and 13 for your stretching exercises. Always stretch before and after all your activities, to warm up and cool down and to prevent injuries from sudden movements.

- Aerobics—Your walking program in Chapter 12 is your initial aerobics program. As you progress, you can alternate walking with running, jogging, and aerobic dancing. To get the full cardiovascular benefits, you gradually work up to the goal of a thirty-minute aerobic session three times a week.
- Strength training—The weight-lifting program in Chapter 13 is my favorite form of strength training. Use the routine suggested in that chapter, or modify it as needed. You can also use calisthenics, aerobics, and sports to increase your strength. For maximum benefit, you should include strength training three times a week.
- Sports and recreation—These activities, discussed in Chapter 14, amplify your fitness program and teach you how to have fun. Try to play as often as you can.

To get total physical conditioning and as an alternative to the walking program, some of my clients start out with my favorite stationary bicycle, the Lifecycle, the biggest boon to cardiorespiratory fitness that I have encountered. Lifecycles are excellent for burning calories. The Lifecycle has a self-contained computer program that allows you to progress toward fitness while monitoring your condition. Strive for thirty-minute workout sessions.

The program is designed to increase your fitness level, lower your resting heart rate, build stamina, and improve your circulatory system. You can find Lifecycles in your local health club or buy one from a sports equipment store. Any exercise bicycle will help produce the same results if you learn to use it properly and monitor your heart rate.

My clients start their workouts with five minutes on the Lifecycle, building up to a target goal of thirty minutes, three times a week. They do five minutes of basic stretches to develop their strength and flexibility. They then start a beginner's weight-training circuit on the machines, including bench presses, leg presses, sit-ups, leg extensions, lat pull-downs, and leg curls. At the beginning, they do six to eight repetitions for the upper body and ten repetitions for the lower body, in two sets. They end their workout with five minutes of stretching. The entire workout lasts one hour. In addition, they complete a thirty-minute aerobic workout three times a week.

EXERCISE TIPS

You can set up the same kind of program with your Weekly Exercise Worksheet. Start slowly, and build up to a full-fledged program. Use the following tips to help you get started.

- It may seem as if you have to exercise daily to fit in all parts of your program. You don't, and you shouldn't. Daily exercise will increase your risk of injury, particularly when you are a beginner.
- Combine the four parts of your fitness program in various ways to eliminate boredom and fulfill your requirements in three or four workout sessions. Stretch and swim aerobically, or bike aerobically (keeping your heart rate up) to your health club, then do your weight training. Be creative with your combinations.
- Easy does it. As you begin to exercise, take each new step slowly and carefully. Don't try to do a lot of repetitions; concentrate on perfecting your form at first, then build up your repetitions gradually. If you do too much at first, your body will rebel with aches and pains.
- Make sure that you are conditioning the whole body. By cross-training, or including several kinds of exercise in your fitness program, you'll avoid muscle strains and devise a routine that has enough built-in diversity to prevent boredom. The greatest benefit of incorporating a cross-training program is evenly

strengthened muscles. This helps prevent injuries when participating in the sport of your choice.

- When doing your stretching, weight training, and walking,
follow the photographs in this book. Try to work out in front
of a mirror, so you can check your positioning. Proper position
is essential for maximum benefits and for preventing injuries.

- Make sure you have your doctor's OK before starting out with
any exercise program.

- If you can stick to your new RRP Fitness Program three times
a week for two weeks, the chances are you will stick with it
forever. Enthusiasm will carry you through the first week. The
second week, there will be all kinds of alternatives to choose
from. If you stick to this for two weeks, you will notice so
many benefits that you will actually look forward to your
fitness activity.

- One thing for sure, you must have a regular exercise schedule
to stay on track. If you don't, you will never find that "right
time." I look at my exercise time as an appointment I must
keep.

- Try to find an exercise partner to help keep your momentum
going. Make sure that person is as committed to health and
physical fitness as you are.

- You can use little things to make your workouts more
enjoyable. Buy inspirational books. I always read the new
muscle and fitness magazines, especially the latest findings on
nutrition, new philosophies and theories, weight training, and
success stories.

- When you design your program to provide health benefits,
you will find it touches other areas of your life as well. The
key is to hang in there and stay with it.

- Reward yourself in healthy ways. Most of us are accustomed
to rewarding ourselves in unhealthy ways. It can take some
creativity to figure out new ways to reward yourself. But by
listing the healthy things that please you, you will learn more
about yourself and be able to treat yourself well.

REWARDING YOURSELF

At this beginning stage of your recovery, you may not have a lot of money to spend. Believe it or not, this obstacle can enhance your fitness. By participating in my aerobic walking program, which didn't cost a dime, I actually saved the money I would have spent on other activities. Gradually, I saved enough to reward myself with a bike and a health club membership paid for on a monthly basis.

The best way to get "strokes" and support for your courageous effort toward fitness is to find someone to exercise with you. Your exercise partner could be another recovering alcoholic or addict, a family member, or a friend. You could find a number of partners for your various activities—someone to walk with, bike with, or join you at the gym.

Make it a point to find partners who are starting at the same level you are. Set up a schedule to meet regularly and stick to this commitment. In this way, you create a support group to enhance your experience and motivation. But remember, though it is nice to have partners in your fitness program, *you* are ultimately responsible for your fitness program.

SHORT-TERM AND LONG-TERM GOALS

"The courage to change the things I can" certainly plays a big part in your new health program and your commitment to establishing lifelong health habits. You can make changes by setting your goals. Start with the long-term goals of good health and optimum fitness. Most of the people I work with find that setting short-term goals and achieving them is the key to overcoming bad habits. When they reach their short-term goals, they set higher goals. Once they achieve their goals, they strive to maintain what they achieve.

The action of exercise helps people stick to their goals. When they are tired, frustrated, or anxious, they long for the satisfaction of a good workout. They love the release a good workout gives. They enjoy the sensation of endorphins being released, giving them a natural high, so much more pleasant than the high from chemicals. Their new program replaces their need for drugs. They get their highs naturally, if you will. Your successes will feed on each other and build. You will experience self-fulfillment and pleasure and a lifestyle change that will have a tremendous impact on your recovery.

The success of your program and new life depends on how motivated you are. Your mental toughness is the most important ingredient in carrying out this program for the rest of your life. The best way to ensure proper motivation is by learning how to set goals.

Goals will give you direction and allow you to focus your energies and efforts. Goals help you to measure your progress.

Decide what you want. Write it down. (There's a form for this in Appendix A, on pages 226–27.) "Terminal vagueness" is part of the alcoholic's disease and keeps us from sticking to our course of action. We can be easily distracted.

GUIDELINES FOR GOAL SETTING

When you set goals, be as detailed as possible. Specific goals will provide you with more of a challenge and capitalize on your potential. For instance, instead of writing, "I want to increase my cardiovascular fitness," put, "I will follow the aerobic walking program outlined in this book for 30 days." Or if you choose a cycling program, write, "I will work toward riding two to three miles three times a week for approximately 20 to 30 minutes." This allows you to set a specific goal that is easy to measure.

Visualize how you want to look. Create a picture of what you expect to accomplish. Picture yourself taking 20 seconds off your jogging time, or imagine the feeling of a finish-line tape stretching across your chest as you finish first in a 10K run. Imagine the feelings of being a winner in life again. Remember: "You can do it if only you believe you can!"

Make sure your goals are realistic. Ego and grandiosity can defeat you right here. In all your humility, set a moderate goal.

Make sure that it will challenge you and push you to improve. If you succeed in these moderate goals, you will gain the confidence to elevate your expectations, which will lead to further success. By experiencing "mini" success, you will build your confidence. The results will be increased self-esteem and appreciation of your abilities.

Outline your plan to reach your desired goal. Break every long-term goal into smaller objectives. These small steps will be the stairs you climb to reach your desired goals. The danger of long-range goals is the lack of opportunity to reward yourself. When you reach your short-term goals, your opportunities for success are greater.

Now that you have set up your timetable, you should have a definite plan to meet that goal. To have your plan work, you must work your plan. Concentrate your energies on pursuing your goals. Believe in your success. Picture your body being healed from the inside out. Be persistent and be "willing to go to any lengths" to reach your goals. Within you lies the power to obtain whatever you want. You can achieve your goals. Just believe in yourself! Place this statement in front of you: "Day by day in every way, I am becoming more successful."

Review your progress and applaud yourself as you achieve each goal. Make sure you retest yourself and take your measurements. This helps you stay on track and allows you to make any changes that your program may require.

Place your goals on the mirror in your bathroom and on your refrigerator door. This not only programs your subconscious but constantly reminds you to stay on track.

NO INSURMOUNTABLE BARRIER

We desperately need this goal-setting procedure. We must instill some form of discipline into our previously undisciplined lives. This process will keep you motivated. Someone who doesn't have a plan or goal is like a ship without a rudder. Goals help you by giving direction to setting up your own health care program. They allow you to experience a feeling of accomplishment. You will be ensuring success as you journey toward your ultimate goal of a healthy life.

The checklists, personal inventories, and worksheets, and other forms of self-evaluation in this book are used for self-measurement. They help you set up and meet your short- and long-term goals. These worksheets, the tests to assess your level of fitness strength and flexibility, and the worksheets for detecting stress will help you discover the solutions and changes you need in order to enrich and maintain your sobriety. You will then be able to apply the ideas in this book with more meaning for your recovery. You can begin to work on areas that need to be changed, learn to accept the things you cannot change, and have the wisdom to know the difference. These worksheets, quizzes, and lists are to be used as guides to chart your way toward sanity and wellness.

To conclude this chapter, here is one of my favorite sayings from Ralph Waldo Emerson: "There is no defeat except from within. There is really no insurmountable barrier save your own inherent weakness of purpose."

ASSIGNMENTS

1. Fill out your Weekly Exercise Worksheet. Give yourself plenty of time to review all of Part Two, and time to practice and learn which forms of exercise you enjoy most. Don't work out every day; three or four times a week is enough.
2. Fill out your Goals for Health Worksheet and post it where you can see it frequently.
3. Find a "fitness buddy," preferably on your fitness level, to join you.
4. Find a picture of what you expect to look like and put it on the refrigerator door.

PART III
STRESS AND SUCCESS

Yesterday is but a dream,
Tomorrow is only a vision.
But today well lived makes
Every yesterday a dream of happiness,
And every tomorrow a vision of hope.
Look well, therefore, to this day.

FROM THE SANSKRIT

16
The Monster Called Stress

*W*hen we are newly sober, our coping skills are minimal at best. In our drinking days, we tried to solve our frustrations, struggles, interpersonal and financial difficulties, anger, fear, resentments, and loneliness by taking chemicals. We drank too much, popped too many pills, snorted coke, or shot up—anything to numb these daily stressful occurrences. At the same time, the symptoms of our disease eroded the foundations of our lives.

In the past, we were haunted by fears that our best wasn't good enough. Somehow we just couldn't measure up. Paralyzed by these fears, we performed inadequately, thus validating our fears. We felt the need to cover up our insecurities by cheating, lying, and not facing up to responsibilities, or by playing the big shot. This led us to further alienate those around us. The combination of our stresses and addictions forced us to hit rock bottom physically and emotionally.

BEGIN WITH AWARENESS

Your first step in managing stress is to view yourself from a new perspective. You need to learn skills for healthy living and develop more self-awareness. You must learn how you create stress, how to become aware of the stress in your work and personal life, and how to listen to your body and mind when they signal the need for change. You need to evaluate the role stress plays in relation to your mental and physical fitness.

It is important to know that we generate our own stress by the way we react to our environment. Before recovery, we looked at our world with "rose-colored glasses" or, on the other end of the scale, with a sense of impending doom.

Fear of failure takes time to disappear. Eliminating your addictions won't solve your problems, but a realistic self-awareness will provide the confidence to participate in a new health care program and strive to meet your goals.

Two major areas of stress are on your job and in your personal life. What stresses are you experiencing now? Have you been fired due to your addiction? Is an intimate relationship going through a crisis? If you are faced with problems in both areas, you have a tremendous amount of stress in your life.

The 12-step program in A.A. helps us restructure our thinking, which in turn aids us in overcoming life's daily stresses. In A.A., our first step is to admit we have lost control over our lives and need to gain humility. We have to get rid of anger and resentments and learn how to forgive others, as well as ourselves. We begin to clean up the "wreckage of our past" and ask our Higher Power to help us. We go to our meetings and get a sponsor. Slowly we recognize that success in sobriety depends on our self-involvement and spiritual focus. Our stress levels decrease because we are no longer fighting ourselves. We view life in terms of service instead of self-seeking actions. We learn to love ourselves and then love others we are connected to. This is a gradual process, one that has to be renewed daily.

By learning to adapt the steps of A.A. to all parts of our lives, we can learn the skills that make recovery more comfortable, particularly when we are faced with the stressful areas in our lives.

EFFECTS OF STRESS

First, consider what kinds of physical damage are caused by stress and why you need to decrease your stress to increase your physical and mental health. Understanding the symptoms of stress will make you more aware of the stress in your life. Some of the damaging effects of stress are given in the following lists.

Physical Effects. Left unchecked, responses to stress lower resistance to diseases in vital organs and can lead to death. These responses include:

- Increased blood glucose, heart rate, and blood pressure
- Shortness of breath
- Numbness, tingling, and coldness in hands and feet
- Stomach upsets and gastrointestinal disorders
- Tight, rigid muscles
- Low-back pain
- Headaches
- Dry mouth
- Heavy perspiration

Emotional Effects. Stress has many emotional effects as well:

- Anxiety
- Anger
- Boredom
- Depression
- Fatigue
- Frustration

- Irritability
- Low self-esteem
- Compulsive worrying
- Tension
- Defensiveness

Mental Effects. Some mental effects of stress are:

- Poor concentration
- Poor memory
- Poor performance

Behavioral Effects. Stress is evidenced by behavior that includes:

- Overeating
- Drug and alcohol abuse
- Restlessness
- Isolation
- Poor sleep habits

Occupational Effects. On the job, stress shows up in the form of:

- Job burnout
- Poor work performance
- Accidents
- Inability to cooperate with co-workers
- Frequent absences
- Frequent use of health and disability insurance

After reviewing this list, you can understand how stress affects every area of your life. The toll it takes on you physically and mentally can increase the risk of poor health.

FITNESS: A SOUND MIND PLUS A HEALTHY BODY

You need to be aware of your various physical and emotional responses to stress. How do you handle situations? How does your body respond? What is going on in your mind? How do you feel, and what do you do to meet those feelings?

Fitness requires a sound mind combined with a healthy body. The two must communicate adequately for you to achieve your true potential. A sound mind can't achieve desirable actions unless the body is physically capable of carrying out what the mind is planning. A trained, vibrant body can't achieve peak performance unless the brain can send its messages along the proper path.

You must learn to recondition your thinking and apply your Recovery/Relapse-Prevention Program to combat the stresses in your life. As a form of preventive medicine, you need to keep these stresses from occurring.

YOU DESERVE SUCCESS

An integral part of recovery is learning that you deserve success and all the good things of life that you are entitled to. With the components of this program, along with your A.A. program, therapy, and any other forms of support you need in the recovery process, you will have the strength to confront reality without drinking and using drugs.

A big plus of the RRP Program is that it forces you to be involved with others who are helping themselves. The changes you need to make will be possible when you see you are not alone. If you decide to join a gym or cycling group or a bowling team, you will see others strive and succeed and fail, and come back and try again. This creates energy that spurs you on.

When you see other people achieve the things you want and know what they went through to succeed, you become motivated to accept the same challenges. You can read success stories every day. Television talk shows are filled with guests with success stories. Now more than ever, famous people from all parts of society are coming forth with stories concerning their battles and triumphs over various forms of addiction. You can help eliminate failure by believing their example and feeling the inward motivation to forge ahead.

Self-healing begins with making your own decisions about going to any lengths to restore your health. You can recapture what you thought you had lost in body, mind, and spirit. You *can* heal yourself.

We have all decided that we want to live, not die—to be healthy, not sick. Our preventive approach can make the difference between a depressed, sick life or a vital, fulfilling one. Now that you are sober and free, you are not expected to live life as though it were a prison sentence. You are entitled to a quality life of sobriety. You can achieve your potential for good health. That is what this section of the book is designed to do.

ASSIGNMENTS

1. When you catch yourself worrying or expecting the worst, relax and imagine positive events and make positive statements. (I deserve this. . . . I expect the best.)
2. Make a list of your assets on two 3 × 5 cards. Place one on a bathroom mirror, and carry the other one with you. Read the list out loud to yourself three times a day.
3. Treat yourself to a daily catnap.
4. Take a break and do some stretches to release your tension buildup.
5. Treat yourself to a brisk walk around the block.

17
Your Stress
Assessment

I have often heard my fellow addicts say, "If I had not been on drugs or booze, the stress I was going through at the time would have killed me!"

The more I discovered the physiological damage caused by stress, the more I recognized the foolishness of that statement. Research shows that the cause of stress is your body's inability to respond appropriately to its signals. By drinking to escape from our problems, we were not only poisoning our bodies, but we were also, in a sense, aiding and abetting disease. We were practicing skills for acquiring sickness. Now we can learn healthy living skills with the help of A.A.'s 12 Steps and the Recovery/Relapse-Prevention Program.

Newly sober, we must constantly be aware of the dangers of stress. Our bodies and minds can't tolerate the stresses other people seem able to handle. We need to know what is causing our stresses before we can do anything about them. We need to develop a new awareness of ourselves and develop new skills for coping with the stresses of sobriety.

151

When we were drinking, our response to stress was overreaction. We were constantly tossed about through the storms of life, "victims of circumstances" with little or no control. Today you are sober, and your life has changed dramatically. Now you need to learn how to respond by changing yourself.

You have the choice to make this change and respond to life's pressures in new and innovative ways. It is never too late to learn these new skills. When pressures build in sobriety, you don't have to push the panic button and react. You have the ability to plan alternate escape routes, with new and different ways to cope with your stresses.

YOUR STRESS ASSESSMENT

Hundreds of biochemical changes occur every time you are under stress. Your fight-or-flight response can cause fatigue, headaches, palpitations, and other related symptoms. When stress symptoms occur repeatedly over a period of time, these responses are generally known as psychosomatic symptoms.

The Stress Assessment form in Appendix A (pages 229-30) will give you an idea of the types, frequency, and varying degrees of symptoms of stress you suffer from. This chart will make you more aware of the stresses in your life. Believe me, before I started charting my program, I had no idea what was setting off my colitis and headaches. I soon found out that it was a crowded environment, among other stress-related situations. When I became aware of my physiological symptoms, I was motivated to find out how to pinpoint those areas of my life and start to work on them to alleviate a stressful lifestyle.

The key to managing your stress is understanding the unique stress patterns in your life. Patterns triggering reactions to stress vary tremendously from person to person. The more you observe your feelings before, during, and after stressful situations, the better able you will be to understand how stress affects your everyday life.

The best way to beat stress is with the game plan outlined in this book. First find out what stresses are occurring now. Then keep a daily record in a stress detection log. The daily log will reveal the patterns of stress in your life. When you analyze your stress and how it affects your body and behavior, you will be ready to start your own stress management program.

Look over the Stress Assessment list and check the physical and mental signs of stress you suffer from. You may want to add to this list, since people have individual responses to stress.

When you have completed the checklist, go back and study your yes responses. Learn to detect your personal stress signals.

YOUR DAILY STRESS DETECTION LOG

Using the form in Appendix A (page 232), make a Daily Stress Detection Log. Whenever you feel upset, distressed, angry, pressured, anxious, panicked, or frustrated, write in your log. Explore each event. How do you react to the situations that come up? How does your body respond? What are you feeling? Feelings may be what you have suppressed the most. You must learn to recognize fear, anger, jealousy, envy, greed, restlessness, loneliness, and other kinds of feelings. Write them down. Your log will help you look at your life in sobriety, cope with its stresses, and stop feeling like a victim. Your degree of success will be directly related to how often you write in your log.

When you were faced with a stressful situation, think of how you responded. What was the trigger? How did you think? More importantly, how did you feel? How did others respond to your reaction? How effective was your response? What were the negative effects this incident had on you? When you answer these questions, you will develop more self-awareness and come closer to discovering the many facets and possibilities in each situation.

After you analyze each event, patterns will be obvious. Later, you can generalize and ask yourself some important questions. This will speed up your self-analysis of your stress. For instance, ask:

• How frequently do I experience stressful events each day?

- How distressing are these occurrences to me?
- Are these events expected, or are they surprises?
- What keeps me from expressing my feelings (fear of rejection, fear I will experience some kind of loss)?
- What would I say if I could express myself?
- What other ways could I release the tension generated by these feelings?

Few people are used to evaluating their behavior like this, so it may take time to be able to "tune in" to the messages your body and mind send you. When you log your reactions every day, you will be able to use your observations to cope with the stressful events in your life. Remember, this is a day-at-a-time program!

ASSIGNMENTS

1. Complete your Stress Assessment.
2. Go over the list with your doctor to be sure these symptoms are not caused by illness.
3. Start keeping your Daily Stress Detection Log.

18
Stress and Sobriety

Successful recovery, from a psychological point of view, depends on learning to actively overcome discomfort about life's many problems. Everyone has psychological problems that compound the stresses of life. Our alcohol and drug abuse has affected us mentally and emotionally. We have developed negative attitudes and have convinced ourselves that we are no good and worth less than others. We know deep down inside how "different" we are and that nobody really understands us. We have been told we suffer from "terminal uniqueness." We withdraw more as the stresses of our life build.

HELP FOR PSYCHOLOGICAL PROBLEMS

At this stage you need to treat your psychological problems. The best treatment I have found is to go to A.A. meetings and talk with my A.A. sponsor. Therapy with a qualified professional can be of enormous value. I also believe in a Higher Power, whom I choose to call God. None of us can survive and handle the daily stresses of life alone.

155

I was under tremendous stress during my first week of sobriety. I was evicted, had my checking account closed, had my phone disconnected, and had my car repossessed. Every day, I went to A.A. meetings, where I found fellow addicts who understood what I was going through and offered me a great amount of solace and relief. My stress level dropped immediately. The sharing in meetings helped me to see my problems more clearly. Then I could take the appropriate action to solve my problems and eliminate the stress they were causing. I was advised to trust a Higher Power, go to meetings, read the "Big Book," get a sponsor, and "clean house."

I met a wonderful woman in A.A. named "Boston Helen." Boston Helen used to say, "Put the plug in the jug," and, "You won't get drunk if you don't take that first drink." She told me that whenever I felt uncomfortable and crazy, I should get to a meeting—immediately—and share what I was going through. I was always amazed at the magic I felt when I opened up and revealed my pain. In return I received support, advice, and encouragement.

To this day, I leave A.A. meetings with an extra lift in my spirit and a better attitude about life. Yes, A.A. and the 12 Steps are important elements in keeping me sober. Through them, I changed my negative attitude to a positive one and included a spiritual direction in my life. It worked for me, and it can work for you.

FACING YOUR FRUSTRATIONS

Alcoholics are like little babies; we want what we want when we want it. We feel, just like babies, that the world should revolve around us. When we were drinking and faced frustrations, we would blow up, scream, cry, throw things, or lash out at those we loved. We never expressed this behavior when we were sober, because of our insatiable need for love and our tremendous fear of rejection. So we buried our hurt and resentful feelings. When resentments grow, we face a tremendous temptation to escape from our psychic pain with alcohol or drugs.

There is a solution to our resentments in the 12 Steps of A.A. In

Step 4, we get all our resentments down on paper and forgive others and ourselves for each and every resentment. We list the person, place, or thing we feel resentment toward. We decide what parts of our lives—financial, emotional, sexual, interpersonal—are affected by our resentments. We list the character defects that play a part in our resentments. Was it greed, lust, pride, envy, egomania?

Almost all of my resentments came from a self-centered fear. After I wrote down every resentment, from childhood on, I shared this list with my A.A. sponsor, prayed, and experienced a tremendous sense of freedom. What I had pictured as an arduous endeavor turned out to be my gateway to freedom and love. My years of bottled-up anger and frustration melted away. My attitude about life changed as I entered the "fourth dimension" that the Big Book of A.A. talks about.

SOBRIETY AND STRESS

As you acquire a positive mental attitude through what you learn in A.A., your stress will diminish rapidly. You will start gaining self-confidence and using the "action" habit to solve your problems. You will not be coddled in any self-imposed "pity parties." As you practice the principles of A.A. each day, your life will get much better. Life may get so good that you enter the danger zone of complacency, which can lead you back to the bottle. But if you discipline yourself and stick with your RRP program and diaries, you will constantly be challenged to grow.

If you don't consistently program your mind with positive thought patterns, the old thought patterns and habits will eventually return. These old patterns lie dormant in the dark recesses of your mind just like weeds wanting to grow through the patches of new grass. Negative attitudes develop "stinkin' thinking."

Sobriety is stressful because it constitutes a major change in your life. You will grieve over the loss of your closest companions—alcohol and drugs. Loneliness and fear can tempt you to return to your addictions. You get rid of these "needs" by using the techniques described in this chapter.

Your first year of sobriety should be spent growing physically, mentally, and spiritually. This is where your energies need to be focused. At the beginning of your second year, you will slowly start making long-range plans that will change your life dramatically—for the better. Your self-confidence and new self-awareness will aid you in making positive changes in your life.

SOBRIETY, STRESS, AND WORK

Most of us have job problems caused by rebellion against authority, self-centered fear, and immense feelings of insecurity. Most jobs include expectations, duties, and interpersonal relationships. By your very perceptions of and reactions to each of these areas, you have the choice to become a victim or victor. You will naturally encounter stressful situations over which you have no control, but, by and large, you modify your stresses within your own mind.

As you develop experience in coping and growth, you become capable of making quality decisions about the directions you want your life to take. You will make decisions about your occupation and relationships. Hopefully, you will seek a job that gives you satisfaction and fulfillment, rather than money alone or the approval of your mate, family, or society.

I had to come to grips with the job decision after my first year of sobriety. Before I got sober, I left teaching because I felt it could not support me and my children. I didn't take the time to see how I could apply my skills to other areas that I loved. I just wanted a profession in which I could make lots of money. I was very successful, but I was not satisfied.

When I got to the recovery home, I was so confused about everything that I couldn't make any decisions. I didn't even know who I was. I kept asking myself, "What am I going to do? How am I going to support myself?" As my mind cleared and my body recuperated, I slowly started on a program of self-discovery. I vowed not to subject myself to the stresses created by a job that made me miserable. I realized that if I didn't decide what to do in this area of my life, my sobriety would be at stake. Gradually, I realized I could combine my background in physical education and love of sports with my experience as an alcoholic. The work that came out of that realization has made me happier than any other work I have ever done.

I am not asking you to quit your job, only to examine it. How can you improve your circumstances in your job? Maybe you don't have to change your job—only your attitude.

SOBRIETY, STRESS, AND MONEY

Alcohol and drugs wreak havoc with our financial security. They demand high prices at low wages as they fuel our spending and curb our earning ability.

While we were addicted, our financial problems and our attitudes toward money corresponded directly to our massive fears. We became greedy and full of false pride. We treated money irresponsibly, compounding our financial problems and impairing our relationships at home and on the job. Many of us have debts that seem impossible to pay.

If you are severely in debt or still unemployed, get help. Debtors Anonymous can help you solve your financial problems and resolve to stay out of debt.

SOBRIETY, STRESS, AND RELATIONSHIPS

Our sense of friendship, love, and relationships was distorted by alcohol and drugs. It will take much time and energy to relearn how to relate to others.

Since we all suffered from self-centered fear, we hung on to the people we thought could give us security and love. We smothered and alienated those around us with infantile demands. All of us have "used" the people around us to feed our insatiable egos. We needed some person, place, or thing to lean on. When these people failed us, we got angry and drank at them. We were loaded with vengeful thoughts and retaliated. When we did this, we alienated ourselves even further. We had slowly eliminated any hopes of developing healthy relationships with others. We became marooned in a sea of loneliness. We must swim to shore and heal our psychic wounds.

Through Step 4, A.A. teaches us to examine and share our lives. In order to gain love, companionship, and acceptance, you need to take a personal inventory and review your relationships. To fully benefit from this exercise, it helps to share your findings with another human being—someone who understands you (minister, doctor, A.A. sponsor). Together, you can evaluate the areas that cause your stress and unhappiness, and discuss solutions.

When you do this, you will experience a miraculous healing in your heart and mind. You will no longer feel the excruciating pain of loneliness. You will have chipped away at your pride and ego and discovered the beauty of humility. By sharing with someone else, you are building your bridge back to humanity, defeating the loneliness in your life.

YOUR ATTITUDE INVENTORY

Your Personal Attitude Inventory in Appendix A (pages 233–34) will help you discover the stress points in your life. It will highlight the areas of your life that need to be changed. If you don't attempt to eliminate these cancerous elements, you will probably never discover the peace and serenity needed to stay clean and sober.

The questions reveal your general attitudes and style of thinking. By checking the column beside each question that best describes your experiences, you will find the patterns that are the basis for your frustration and stress. You will discover how you "talk" to yourself and what you assume. You may find that your mind is filled with anger and a sense of injustice.

Stress is caused by how you relate to the world. You can reduce the stress in your life by changing your attitudes and perceptions. You can eliminate negative beliefs and expectations, and find other ways to relate. When you do this, you discover what true freedom is. Your negativity no longer has power over you. If you don't get rid of stressful areas, you will surely drink.

It is very hard to change your inner view of yourself and others. You may be holding on for dear life to defenses and behaviors created when you were a child. People with alcoholic patterns have generations of attitudes to overcome. But it is possible to understand your frustrations and fears. It is possible to decrease your isolation and defensiveness. You can manage your stresses and live with happiness.

ASSIGNMENTS

1. Start working on your fourth step—refer to the Big Book of A.A.
2. Share your Personal Attitude Inventory with your A.A. sponsor.
3. Repeat the following affirmations upon arising and before you go to bed at night. As you say these, visualize your affirmations becoming a part of your life. Experience yourself changing. Add to this list from your own self-knowledge.

   • I will let go of my anger.
   • I forgive those I am resentful against.
   • I will accept what I can't change.
   • I am strong and healthy.
   • I thank God for a second chance.
   • I am a winner.

4. Buy an inspirational A.A. tape and listen to it while you are driving. Listen to self-improvement programs.
5. Stick with the winners. Don't run around with negative people. These are time wasters. Stick with people who share your values and goals.

19
Reducing Your Stress

*W*hen you are unable to manage the stress in your life, you open the door to myriad physical and psychological problems. Often, your emotions are your strongest signals that your health and sanity are in danger. Anger, depression, self-hatred, worry, frustration, irritability, and moodiness are the emotional symptoms of stress.

Some forms of stress are not negative. Their symptoms include excitement, nervousness, and elation. A new job, a public-speaking engagement, a first date are all stressful, whether you are sober, drunk, or drugged. But they can be stressful in a positive way. Stress becomes negative and harmful when it continues over long periods of time, creating confusion and despair. As recovering alcoholics with obsessive minds, we can hold on to negative thinking and let our stressed-out emotions rule our lives.

UNDERSTANDING ANGER

Anger is the most disabling emotion we have. It can instantly

162

eliminate any serenity we may have acquired. Anger can drive us back to the bottle faster than anything else. We use the alcohol to anesthetize this socially unacceptable feeling. There is one major drawback, however. Alcohol lowers our inhibitions, and our anger is not anesthetized. Our pent-up rage escapes, and we strike out at anyone and anything that may frustrate us. Research shows that at least half of all assaults and homicides are committed under the influence of alcohol or drugs. Other crimes such as vehicular manslaughter, rape, domestic violence, child abuse, and armed robbery are frequently linked to alcohol and drug abuse. Is it any wonder that anger is a dangerous emotion, particularly when combined with alcohol or drugs?

However, anger toward human conditions such as homelessness, poverty, illness, and injustice produces valuable changes, when channeled compassionately. As long as your anger is directed in positive ways, this emotion cannot kill you. But when fed with grudges or resentments, it can tempt you to drink. It can also fill your life with fear, which is often anger's result. Sometimes we don't know why we are afraid; we just know that our fear suddenly overtakes us when we face a certain person, place, or thing. Frustration can also feed and be fed by anger. None of us has a high tolerance for frustration.

Justifiable anger is another slippery emotion that you cannot afford to entertain. No matter how shabbily or unjustly you have been treated, you just can't afford to indulge in this self-destructive feeling. It will certainly lead you back to drinking.

Finding the causes of your anger can help, but it is most important to develop the ability to cope with the feelings anger generates. When you start to feel rage at the simmering point, you can pick up the phone and talk to another A.A. member. You can go to a meeting and share how you feel. You can run around the block, take a swim, or take a nap. Praying the serenity prayer helps. Sometimes, you just can't change a situation, no matter what. So you simply learn to accept the situation, rather than drink or use drugs. If you are in a situation that needs to be changed, you should only try to change it when you are under control and harboring no anger or resentment. Don't ever act out of anger. You will only regret it.

Before you can make any change, you must remember the slogan "first things first." In other words, you must not drink, no matter what. You must place your sobriety first—before your job and your family. If you value your job and family, you must take precautions to save your life. Otherwise, you can't enjoy these gifts.

LEARNING TO MANAGE YOUR EMOTIONS AND STRESS

Stressful emotions can be deadly if they are not recognized or managed positively. Conversely, stress can push you to heights you never dreamt you could achieve. The key is to recognize and understand your emotions and thereby face your stresses. To do so, you must learn to be comfortable with your emotions and manage your stress. The following stress management guidelines can help.

- A great majority of the people I work with find tremendous relief through professional guidance. They work with a therapist who understands addiction and learn about their emotions, their stresses, and their successes.
- Others become involved with a church. Through the structure of religion and the companionship of their peers, they develop strength and peace.
- Yoga, meditation, and self-hypnosis classes teach self-discipline and control and have a relieving, calming influence on many of my clients.
- Exercise is a great stress reducer. It not only reduces anxiety, but can energize you. Exercise also fights depression and diffuses anger. You feel better and look better. Your self-esteem rises, and you feel capable of handling your destiny.
- Acknowledge that it's the little aggravations that get you crazy—not the big catastrophes. It is important to respond to

the major and minor stresses with the appropriate level of emotion, and not to let each frustration drive you over the edge.

- Follow the daily food program outlined in this book. Foods that cause your sugar levels to rise and drop drastically can make you edgy, nervous, and angry.
- Cut down on caffeine. It causes the highs and lows that make people incapable of handling stress.
- Try to set priorities and manage your time. Remember to practice "first things first." List in order of priority the things you want to accomplish each day. You will be amazed at how this will reduce your stress and increase your efficiency.
- Don't be a people pleaser. Just say no. It is not realistic to say yes to every request. If you say yes to other people's requests, you will be kept from taking care of the things you need to accomplish.
- If you make mistakes, don't be overwhelmed. Step back, look at the situation, and see what valuable lesson you can learn from it.

THE POWER OF SLEEP

Not all stress reduction techniques involve hard work. One of the best ways to calm your spirit is through sleep. Sleep helps reduce your stress and heals your body and mind.

You are probably familiar with the saying "The best defense is a good offense." This might sum up the importance of sleep in your battle against stress. Since the brain controls biological survival, you need to nourish it through rest and sleep. If you don't get a good night's rest, you will face the day irritable, tired, grouchy, and unable to cope. When you are in this state, your ability to cope with any stresses will be minimal. If you continue to have sleep disturbances, you will become physically and mentally exhausted and experience great anxiety. It will also become increasingly difficult to concentrate, and you will become depressed.

A lot of my clients ask me how much sleep they need. I tell them to function well, they need at least six to eight hours of uninterrupted sleep. If you have trouble getting to sleep now, when you start your exercise program, you will get a good night's sleep.

When I first became sober, I used to wake up in a startled, agonized state after dreaming vividly about drinking and being found drunk. I mentioned these dreams in an A.A. meeting and found that many others had had the same experience. I found that by increasing the number of meetings I attended, I could eliminate these dreams. I am always grateful to wake up sober. I love feeling rested and refreshed—no hangover, no guilt, no worrying about whether I hit someone with my car during the night.

It can take a while for your nervous system to adapt to a regular night's sleep, but you should not take sleeping medications. Your goal is a healthy, drug-free sleep. You need to develop sleep patterns that build the energy reserves needed to cope with the various stresses of sobriety. Here are some pointers to help you sleep:

- Eat a light meal at dinnertime. You don't want your stomach working overtime when you are trying to sleep.
- Limit any fluids for at least two hours before your bedtime. Arising in the middle of the night to go to the bathroom will disturb a good night's sleep.
- Sleep on a firm, comfortable mattress.
- Make sure your sleeping environment is quiet. Get rid of noisy clocks, banging heaters, and creaking doors.
- Go to bed with the intention of going to sleep. Don't watch TV or listen to music while you're in bed; the sounds can interfere with your sleep.
- Make sure your drapes or shades are dark enough to shield your sleeping area from morning and night lights.
- Your room temperature should be around 68 degrees.
- Mentally, approach bedtime with a positive attitude. Know that you have done all you can do for today and look forward to tomorrow.

• Read, listen to soft music, talk with your mate, or take a warm bath before you go to bed. If you develop a relaxing routine, you will be much calmer and get to sleep more easily. Whatever routine you adopt, make sure it is relaxing and not arousing. Make sure that the material you choose to read or listen to is not frightening or depressing.

TAKE A BREAK

To truly curb stress and negative emotions, you should learn to give yourself relaxation breaks throughout the day. Research shows that people who include breaks during work have fewer illnesses. Employers must give their workers breaks, which are usually used for drinking coffee, smoking cigarettes, and eating sugar. This kind of break further drains the body of energy.

If you use your break to relax, using a form of meditation, self-hypnosis, or visualization, you will come away from your break time energized. You should try to get outside or change your environment to aid you in this energizing process.

EXERCISE

If you want to enjoy a quality sobriety with minimal stress, exercise is mandatory in helping you relieve your tension. It acts the same way on your body as sleep does. It can restore your energy. Through cardiovascular and respiratory conditioning and the development of muscle strength, you can reduce stress—even prevent it. Your exercise program will return to you the self-esteem you have lost. You will experience control over your life. I tell my clients the human brain can concentrate on only one thing at a time. When you exercise, you have little time to worry. If you want to regain your self-respect, taking care of your physical body is mandatory. You need a strong body to survive the impact stress has in your life.

Stress management in sobriety is necessary to keep you from taking that first drink. Not only do these techniques help you stay sober, but they provide you with your own preventive medicine program.

ASSIGNMENTS

1. Reward yourself daily in some way.
2. Treat yourself to a massage.
3. Find a place where you can scream for a couple of minutes.
4. Take a class in yoga, meditation, self-hypnosis, or relaxation.

20
The Road to
Self-Respect

Congratulate yourself. Applaud. Pat yourself on the back. You have made the commitment to a healthy lifestyle. You are dramatically altering your recovery. You have reduced your chances of returning to alcohol and drugs for relief.

If you worked on your program as you read through this book, you are probably beginning to feel healthy, strong, and hopeful. You have learned that you must update your lifestyle with fitness, nutrition, stress management, and a strong spiritual belief. You have acquired a precious asset—self-respect.

Maybe you found some of the worksheets or assignments discouraging, but you thought about them anyway. You gave yourself the gift of self-knowledge.

By exercising, you have sweated out those poisonous toxins lying dormant in your body. Your skin and hair have a healthy glow, and your head is clear. By combining fitness and nutrition, you have no doubt begun to lose that bloated look caused by abuse. Your eyes are clear and bright. You are losing weight and gaining compliments. By adding knowledge about stress and success, you are beginning to exhibit the poise under stress you so often yearned for. You are starting to like yourself and can accept and love others. Because of your A.A. meetings and other support groups, you will never again know the horrible pain of loneliness. You have learned that there is a kind, caring, and loving Higher Power who will never let you down.

You will feel more and more confident as you grow accustomed to the control you have over your life. Each success will motivate you to stick with your new RRP Program.

The best motivation of all is to keep in mind that you have an incurable, potentially lethal disease. You know you must live without alcohol.

You don't have to be ashamed of this disease. It is not your fault. You didn't wake up one morning and say, "I think I will become an alcoholic." You did not choose to suffer from this disease.

Yes, you did things that caused you great guilt and suffering because you were sick. Now you know the difference. You no longer have to wonder what is wrong with you. You have recognized you have a threefold disease—physical, mental, and spiritual. Your first and most important step is to recognize that you are powerless over alcohol, and abstinence is your only answer. Then, you learn to rebuild yourself. Once you apply your RRP Program to your new life, you will not want the "old you" back again. You will respect your health and happiness too much to destroy them.

AFFIRMING YOUR SUCCESS

You may feel threatened by your success. As children, many of us lived under enormous expectations. We felt pressured to achieve unrealistic goals. Our goals became so high that any moderate success may have been viewed as failure. We were devastated if we were not Number 1 and did not meet our parents' or others' expectations. We learned somehow, through all of this, that people don't value us for who we are, but for what we do.

This may be twisted thinking, but it is an attitude that the majority of us carry into our adult lives. Most of us seem to have grown up with an inner voice that is critical—the voice of parents, teachers, and our low self-esteem. A.A. circuit speaker Bob E. calls these voices "the committee." The committee takes away any feeling of success and places us under constant pressure.

Think about it—how do you talk to yourself? Does your committee expect the impossible? Turn to the page labeled Your Committee's Criticisms in Appendix A (page 235), and write down the ways you criticize yourself. Use the words you use in your head—all the *shoulds*, the rules, the absolutes, the curses and put-downs. When you are done, read what you've written objectively. Would you talk this way to someone else, expect others to perform so perfectly? Does your committee have any useful suggestions, or is it relentlessly critical and abusive? It is time to beat this negative force in your life.

Instead of listening to your committee, write compliments to yourself. There's a section for this on page 235 also. Forget the criticisms; concentrate on your good qualities. Learn to evaluate your positive self; let the committee be the childish critic. Whenever you experience the committee trying to put you down, make a list that builds you up. Write down the good things you would like to experience. Leave this list in a place where you can see it, and repeat these messages at frequent intervals during the day. You will soon discover an improvement in your self-respect.

When you list positive statements (affirmations) to get rid of negative thought patterns, you uproot the dysfunctional attitudes that perpetuate the negative aspects of your life. If you repeat positive statements often enough, you program your subconscious to encourage a positive reality. Your behavior and feelings project these inner attitudes.

Affirmations and positive thoughts are not meant to fabricate magic in your world. Grandiose thoughts can be as destructive as critical ones. Affirmations help us view the real world positively and eliminate frustrating thoughts and beliefs. To help eliminate your negative attitudes, practice affirmations such as those listed here. Add to the list in Appendix A as you think of new affirmations.

- I believe I am a special human being.
- I am a possibility thinker.
- I am entitled to have abundance in my life.
- I can handle my problems with help.
- Today is fantastic. Something wonderful is going to happen.
- I thank my Higher Power and myself for keeping me clean and sober.
- I am a success.
- I take time to appreciate nature.
- I can change unpleasant situations.
- I do have control over the events in my life.

ASSERTING YOUR SELF-RESPECT

When we enter recovery, we can take off the sign we wear around our neck that reads "Kick Me." Our self-esteem is so low that we are almost afraid of our shadow. We suffer such tremendous guilt over how we behaved when we were deranged by chemicals. We are in such need of love that rejection, whether real or imagined, is too debilitating for us to handle. We find ourselves in tremendous turmoil when we have to stand up for ourselves and express our needs and wants.

Assertion Skills. You need to develop assertion skills to get what you want in your personal and professional lives. You have to learn how to work with others; you need other people in your life. You can't expect to get all you need by yourself, or indirectly from others.

You have to get rid of your pride and embarrassment and be able to ask others for help. If your feelings get in your way and keep you from asking, you cut yourself off from your sources. Often, people can't ask for help because they don't know how. It takes certain skills to be able to ask for what you need without being demanding. The ideal way to assert yourself is to stand up for your rights without ignoring the rights of others. You don't have to get angry to be assertive.

The ideal outcome of assertiveness is to make both people winners. The idea is to work out a plan of action that results in an agreeable solution for all involved. Assertiveness takes practice. For practice, try the following experiment. Eventually you will learn that you don't have to be a people pleaser to the extent that you lose your self-respect. You can be more assertive, get the things you deserve, and make friends in the process.

An Experiment in Assertiveness. First, pick an area of your life you have consciously avoided. Make sure it is an area that is causing you discomfort but is not excruciatingly painful. Write down the problem. Note who is involved, how this situation bothers you, your fears, and your desired outcome. Make sure you have a clearcut goal.

Examine the problem from the other person's side, listing how he or she might be thinking and feeling. Set an appointment with that person, allowing enough time for both of you to consider and discuss your alternatives and objectives.

Before you meet, practice telling the other person how you feel. Don't throw the blame on the other individual. Give him or her credit, and isolate your feelings from the other person's behaviors. It helps to write your script ahead of time and read it to your A.A. sponsor or a friend who can be objective about the situation. Have this person give you feedback on your technique.

You should be able to anticipate the responses of the other person before you confront the situation. Don't forget to clarify your rights, and stay on track. It's common to lose the point, and the objective, by rambling off on some emotional tangent. Practice communicating your point of view clearly in various situations.

Meet with the person involved with your problem. Explain what you are trying to do. Say what you have planned to say, then listen as closely as you can to the response. Concentrate on the process rather than the outcome. You may not reach a decision or solution. You can try again.

After your meeting, review the conversation by yourself and with your sponsor. Keep practicing.

THE IMPORTANCE OF SELF-RESPECT

Recovery demands self-respect. Addicts feel afraid and victimized. Those feelings have most likely nagged at you as you achieved sobriety. Enough is enough, don't you think?

Congratulate yourself for being willing to read through this book. You are in the process of compiling a positive profile of the "new you." By completing the evaluations outlined in this book, you can clearly see the things you want to change in your life. When you write down desired results and visualize what you aspire to be, you are participating in a creative process. You are looking at life in a new way that will make it more comfortable.

Yes, you are taking a risk when you try to change your old ideas and behaviors. Unless you are willing to make these changes and to try to learn new ways of living, your recovery will be seriously hampered.

I hope you take the challenges outlined in this book. You are at the beginning of a healthy, joyous, and energizing life in sobriety. You have given yourself a second chance—take advantage of it. You deserve it!

ASSIGNMENTS

1. Compile your list of committee criticisms.
2. Compile your list of compliments and good qualities.
3. Read your affirmations and add to the list with familiar terms from A.A., favorite quotes or verses, and items from your own experience. Repeat your affirmations throughout the day.
4. Practice the assertiveness experiment.

21
A Lifetime of Success

You have come to the end of this book, and have put together your own Recovery/Relapse-Prevention Program. You have learned the steps that will work for you and acquired enough knowledge to implement your program on a daily basis. You are beginning to feel control over your life as you administer your own health care plan. The discipline and structure this program requires will carry over into other areas of your life. You will surely experience a strong feeling of self-confidence, the natural by-product of your new regimen.

You must educate yourself in order to have lasting success with this program. This book teaches you to recognize and appreciate the health you are entitled to. You have learned how chemical abuse has affected your body, how your body functions, and how you want to feel. Once you understand these facts, you won't get caught in the never-ending quick-fix approaches to fitness and health.

REVIEWING YOUR RECOVERY

Constant review is necessary as you learn to implement and maintain your RRP Program. Only you are capable of knowing your progress. What have you learned so far? How do you feel? Do you truly understand the elements involved in being fit? Are you capable of integrating these into your new lifestyle?

Your RRP Program Review at the end of Appendix A (pages 237–40) helps you answer those questions, discover the areas you need to work on, and develop an interest in learning more about yourself. In addition, Appendix C is a recommended reading list that can help you explore other areas of your development.

Along with completing your RRP Program Review, it is important to routinely review your skills in nutrition, fitness, stress management, and success. Fill out your evaluations routinely, and compare your answers over time. Keep your notebook current, recording your goals, successes, and feelings. When you review these areas, you are making a lasting commitment to having a quality life in sobriety.

Don't be surprised or discouraged at the difficulties you experience as you replace old habits with new ones. You may find that you progress more slowly than you expected. Remember, "Progress, not perfection," and, "One day at a time." You have to exert some effort and determination as you learn to take responsibility for choosing one action over another. Remember, *you* control your destiny—no one else!

RECOVERING FOR LIFE

Alcoholism and drug addiction are serious illnesses. Most of us who have been alcoholics or addicts have been at death's door, only to be grabbed by the mighty hand of God and given a second chance. We know how we and our loved ones have suffered.

We also know the power of humor. We have learned to laugh at our mistakes and to celebrate our progress. This laughter and applause can be heard frequently inside the A.A. rooms.

You will need to draw on your faith, your suffering, and your humor to succeed with your RRP Program. Some people will be able to implement these changes immediately. Others may want to work on this plan with a close friend, an A.A. partner, or a family member. Others will waver because they can't decide what they need to change or just can't muster up enough energy to motivate themselves.

Don't worry, and don't give up. Change requires two qualities that recovering alcoholics often struggle with—decision and commitment. Don't dart into this willy-nilly. Take time for yourself and your health. It takes attention, concentration, and decisions to make this program work for you.

Judge yourself by your best efforts. If you start out and don't meet your goals exactly as you planned, don't consider yourself a failure. Don't brood or entertain obsessively discouraging thoughts. You are experiencing the process of trial and error as you try to reshape your life. Regroup, and your next attempt will be more successful.

When I work one on one with my clients, I find the methodical approach outlined here works best. I explain why certain things work best for each individual, and demonstrate the techniques they need to learn. After each session, I ask my clients to spend the rest of the week practicing the skills they have learned.

You can use the same process with yourself, using this book. Go through it slowly. Practice one thing at a time. It takes several weeks to master this program.

I hope this book has helped you acknowledge your pain and given you the promise of a better life. I want you to be able to grab on to the promise of happiness and freedom. You will be able to handle the realities of life with a clear mind and a healthy body.

As you progress in your sobriety and your RRP Program, you undoubtedly will come up with new ways to improve your health. Great! Implement them and pass them on.

Those who go out and "do a little research" must not give up hope. Just keep this book as close to you as your Big Book and try to remember that you have a serious illness that can be treated. Don't ever get so discouraged that you give up. If you want to get well, you can. Your road to wellness and sobriety is outlined for you here.

ASSIGNMENTS

1. Complete your RRP Program Review. Share it with your sponsor, fitness buddy, or a friend.
2. Congratulations.

PART IV
APPENDIXES

Appendix A:
Charts and Worksheets

MEASUREMENT CHART

	Week 1	Week 3	Week 5	Week 7	Short-Term Goal	Long-Term Goal
Date						
Height						
Weight						
Upper Arm						
Chest						
Waist						
Hips						
Thighs						
Calves						

DAILY DIET DIARY

Date: _____
Day: _____

	Situation and Mood Before Eating	Caffeine and Sugar Products
Breakfast Time:		
Lunch Time:		
Dinner Time:		
Snack Time:		

SEVEN-DAY MENU PLAN

Breakfast: Choose from the Breakfast Selections, interchanging them according to your tastes.

Recipes: Consult Appendix B for recipes for these and other meals.

Breakfast Selections:

A. ½ cup grapefruit juice (unsweetened)
1 serving hot cereal, ¾ oz. uncooked
1 slice toasted whole-wheat bread
1 tsp. margarine
1 cup skim milk
decaffeinated coffee or tea

B. ½ cup apple juice (unsweetened)
2 scrambled eggs
1 slice toasted whole-wheat bread
2 pieces bacon
4 oz. skim milk
decaffeinated coffee or tea

C. Myers Protein Banana Shake:
1 medium banana, cut into chunks
¾ cup skim milk
2–3 tbsp. protein powder (milk and egg protein base with
*   no sugar or artificial coloring added)*
6 ice cubes
¼ tsp. vanilla extract

Combine all ingredients except ice cubes in blender container; add ice cubes two at a time, blending after each addition until shake is thick and smooth.
Serves 2

Lunch and Dinner Menus:

Day 1

Lunch	*Dinner*
Cheese-and-tomato sandwich: 3 oz. cheddar cheese, 2 slices tomato, 1 tbsp. sugarless mayonnaise, 2 slices whole-wheat bread	Lamb kabobs
	Baked potato, plain
	$\frac{3}{4}$ cup brussel sprouts
Small lettuce and cucumber salad with herb dressing	Yogurt with chopped-up apple
	Decaffeinated coffee/tea
Fruit: 1 orange	
4 oz. skim milk/decaffeinated tea	

Day 2

Lunch	*Dinner*
Tuna sandwich: 3 oz. water-packed tuna mixed with 1 tbsp. sugarless mayonnaise, lettuce, 2 slices tomato, 2 slices whole-wheat bread	3–4 oz. broiled veal chop
	$\frac{1}{2}$ cup steamed broccoli
	Salad with herb dressing
Fruit: 2 apples	$\frac{1}{2}$ cup plain yogurt with $\frac{1}{2}$ cup strawberries
Decaffeinated iced tea	
	4 oz. skim milk/decaffeinated coffee

Day 3

Lunch	*Dinner*
4 oz. tomato juice	3–4 oz. broiled chicken
Ham-and-cheese sandwich: 2 oz. cooked ham, 2 oz. lettuce, 2 slices whole-wheat bread with 1 tbsp. sugarless mayonnaise	4 oz. baked potato with $\frac{1}{4}$ cup plain yogurt with chives
	$\frac{1}{2}$ cup cooked spinach
Fruit: 2 pears	Endive salad/herb dressing
Decaffeinated coffee/tea	1 cup strawberries
	Decaffeinated coffee/tea

Day 4

Lunch	*Dinner*
4 oz. broiled chicken	Baked fish
1 baked potato	½ cup steamed broccoli
Fruit: ½ cup strawberries ½ cup plain yogurt	Raspberry yogurt: 5 oz. plain yogurt mixed with ½ cup fresh raspberries
Decaffeinated iced tea	Decaffeinated coffee/tea

Day 5

Lunch	*Dinner*
Liverwurst sandwich: 4 oz. sugarless liverwurst, 2 slices tomato, lettuce, 1 tbsp. sugarless mayonnaise, 2 slices whole-wheat bread	Vegetable lasagne
	Baked potato
Fruit: 1 pear	Spiced grapefruit: ½ fresh grapefruit sprinkled with cinnamon and browned under the broiler
4 oz. skim milk	Decaffeinated coffee/tea

Day 6

Lunch	*Dinner*
Leftover vegetable lasagne (4–6 oz.)	Tuna casserole, 1 serving
1 slice whole-wheat bread	Salad: 5 oz. lettuce, watercress, tomato, cucumber, onions, herb dressing
Fruit: 1 orange	Fruit: ½ melon
4 oz. skim milk	Decaffeinated coffee/tea

Day 7

Lunch	*Dinner*
Tomato-and-mozzarella salad	Whole-wheat spaghetti with tomato and basil, 1 serving
1 slice whole-wheat bread	
Fruit: 1 apple	Salad: sliced tomatoes, cucumbers, onions, peas, cauliflower, herb dressing
Decaffeinated iced tea	
	$\frac{1}{2}$ oz. blue cheese and 1 pear
	Decaffeinated coffee/tea

Note: Basic nutritional allowances are for adult men and women. Teenagers should add 2 fruits, 3 oz. meat or fish, and 8 oz. of skim milk to each day's meals.

Snack List:

Use unrefined foods for snacks. Avoid snacks that have large amounts of oil, salt, or sugar or snacks that are heavily processed or have artificial ingredients (such as potato chips, salted nuts, and fast foods). Keep healthful snacks with you at all times—in the car, office, and home, to keep you from reaching for something quick and harmful. Include the following in your snack selection:

- Fresh fruit—particularly those that travel well, such as apples, peaches, and pears
- Raw vegetables—carrots, celery
- Popcorn—without salt or butter
- Puffed-grain cereals
- Whole-grain breads and crackers
- Sunflower, sesame, or pumpkin seeds
- Sugarless peanut butter
- Water-packed tuna
- Cold chicken
- Cheddar cheese cubes
- Sugarless juices
- Dry roasted nuts

FOOD CHART

ELIMINATE ALL SUGAR

Meat

Eat Freely	*Eat Sparingly*
Beef, lamb, pork, veal, chicken, duck, turkey, sugarless frankfurters, smoked bacon, smoked ham, sugarless sausage	Cold cuts, pastrami, fried chicken, canned and glazed ham

Fish

Eat Freely	*Eat Sparingly*
All kinds without sugar	Breaded fish, prepared shrimp cocktail, ready-made tuna salad, fish cakes, deviled crabs

Carbohydrates

Eat Freely	*Eat Sparingly*
Oat flour, oatmeal, soy grits, soy flour, wheat germ, brown rice	Rolls, cake, candy, cookies, biscuits, desserts, flour, ice cream, jam, jelly, sugar in any form

Fruit

Eat Freely	*Eat Sparingly*
All fruits except those listed at right	Applesauce containing sugar, bananas, blueberries, cherries, dried and preserved fruit, fruit cocktail with sugar or syrup, grapes, guava, mangos, prunes, watermelon

Vegetables

Eat Freely	Eat Sparingly
Asparagus, bean sprouts, green beans, broccoli, raw cabbage, cauliflower, chicory, cucumbers, lettuce, onions, green and red peppers, sour and dill pickles, potatoes, pumpkin, radishes, snow peas, spinach, summer squash, tomatoes	Baked beans, barley, canned vegetables, corn, frozen vegetables, hominy, lima beans, sweet pickles, sweet potatoes, yams

Fats

Eat Freely	Eat Sparingly
Butter, margarine, sugarless peanut butter, sugarless mayonnaise, cream cheese, sour cream	Butter whipped with honey, imitation dairy products, mayonnaise, prepared salad dressings

Drinks

Eat Freely	Eat Sparingly
Seltzer, club soda, herb teas, decaffeinated coffee, sugarless bouillon, sugarless lemonade, cider, fruit juices (unsweetened), milk, vegetable juices	Diet sodas containing caffeine, lemonade, grape juice, instant tea mix, punch, coffee, chocolate milk, hot chocolate, instant fruit-flavored drinks, breakfast drinks

Seasonings

Eat Freely	Eat Sparingly
Prepared mustard (most brands, yellow or brown), herbs, spices, salt (not iodized), horseradish, sugarless salad dressings, vinegar (white, cider, or herb)	Chili sauce, ketchup, most soy sauces, cocktail sauce, bottled sauces, wine vinegar, prepared dips

SURVIVAL KIT

• Two 3-ounce pull-top cans of tuna packed in water
• Plastic container of sugarless peanut butter
• Fork, knife, spoon, plastic plate, wide-mouth Thermos
• Jar of instant decaffeinated coffee
• Plastic cup, packets of nonfat dry milk
• Herbal tea bags
• Cans or packages of nuts
• Cans of unsweetened fruit juice
• Protein tablets, vitamins

You may want to add some of your favorite nonperishable snacks. You can keep these in a cooler, basket, or lunch box in your car. Your Survival Kit is important to keep around for sugar crashes.

STANDARD WEIGHT TABLE

Men

Height	Small	Medium	Large
5'2"	128–134	131–141	138–150
5'3"	130–136	133–143	140–153
5'4"	132–138	135–145	142–156
5'5"	134–140	137–148	144–160
5'6"	136–142	139–151	146–164
5'7"	138–145	142–154	149–168
5'8"	140–148	145–157	152–172
5'9"	142–151	148–160	155–176
5'10"	144–154	151–163	158–180
5'11"	146–157	154–166	161–184
6'0"	149–160	157–170	164–188
6'1"	152–164	160–174	168–192
6'2"	155–168	164–178	172–197
6'3"	158–172	167–182	176–202
6'4"	162–176	171–187	181–207

Women

Height	Small	Medium	Large
4'10"	102–111	109–121	118–131
4'11"	103–113	111–123	120–134
5'0"	104–115	113–125	122–137
5'1"	106–118	115–129	125–140
5'2"	108–121	118–132	128–143
5'3"	111–124	121–135	131–147
5'4"	114–127	124–138	134–151
5'5"	117–130	127–141	137–155
5'6"	120–133	130–144	140–159
5'7"	123–136	133–147	143–163
5'8"	126–139	136–150	146–167
5'9"	129–142	139–153	149–170
5'10"	132–145	142–156	152–173
5'11"	135–148	145–159	155–176
6'0"	138–151	148–162	158–179

These tables were published in 1983 by the Metropolitan Life Insurance Company. All heights are with shoes: men's weights include 5 and women's include 3 pounds of indoor clothing.

VITAMIN SUMMARY

THE FAT-SOLUBLE VITAMINS

Major Roles	Deficiency Symptoms	Food Sources	RDA	Safe Maintenance Doses for Alcoholics
		Vitamin A		
Essential for proper growth and health of skin, mouth, respiratory passages, digestive and urinary tracts. Needed for building strong bones and teeth and for the light-sensitive pigments in the eye, which allow night vision.	Night blindness; dry, pimply skin; infection of lining cells in the respiratory tract; increased susceptibility to pneumonia and tuberculosis; eye infections; stunted growth.	Vitamin A is "preformed" in animal foods: liver, eggs, whole milk, cream. In plants, the substances called carotenes are converted to active vitamin A in the body. Carotene is found in dark, green, leafy vegetables; broccoli, spinach, kale; and in carrots.	3,000 IU	5,000–10,000 IU (under medical supervision if patient has chronic liver disease)

Vitamin D

		200 IU	400 IU
Necessary for fat absorption and use of calcium and phosphorus; essential for formation and growth of bones and teeth. Contributes to proper functioning of nerves, heart, and blood-clotting mechanisms.	Bones grow soft. Rickets is a vitamin D deficiency disease seen in children: bowed legs, nodules on ribs, malformed teeth. In adults, softening of bones can lead to shortened bones and fractures.	Fortified milk, egg yolks, liver, tuna, salmon, cod liver oil.	

Vitamin E

		12–16 IU	100 IU
Acts as an antioxidant, protecting fatty acids from going "rancid" in the body; a natural anticoagulant; supplies oxygen to the muscles, promoting strength and endurance. Heals scar tissue.	No clearcut vitamin deficiency disease has been defined.	Polyunsaturated fats (safflower, sunflower, wheat-germ oils). Almonds, walnuts, sunflower seeds; asparagus, beet greens, broccoli, leeks, spinach, sweet potatoes; apples, blackberries, pears.	

Vitamin K

Essential for normal blood clotting.	Symptoms are seen in alcoholics with severely damaged livers. Symptoms include bleeding and hemorrhage.	Green leafy vegetables (especially spinach and cabbage), egg yolks, milk, safflower oil. Yogurt, kefir, and acidophilus milk promote manufacture of vitamin K in the intestine.	No RDA, but 300–500 mcg considered safe and adequate.	Supplements not usually required.

THE WATER-SOLUBLE VITAMINS

Vitamin C

Essential for efficient working of the immune system. Fights infections, detoxifies harmful substances, is necessary for the manufacture of collagen, prevents fatty acid oxidation.	Early symptoms include bruising, listlessness, joint pains, poor endurance. Severe deficiency leads to scurvy: bleeding and swollen gums, loose teeth, hemorrhage, extreme weakness, sore arms and legs, abnormal heartbeat, labored breathing.	Fresh fruit, particularly citrus fruits, and fresh vegetables (broccoli, cauliflower, cabbage, peppers).	60 mg	500 mg–1 g

Vitamin B-1 (Thiamine)

Needed to break down and release energy from carbohydrates; contributes to healthy nervous tissue.	Loss of appetite, muscle cramps, fatigue, anxiety, inability to concentrate, depression. Beriberi, the vitamin-deficiency disease of B-1, causes mental confusion, stiff and painful legs, "flabby" heart, and heart failure.	Milk and milk products, organ meats, brewer's yeast, dark green vegetables, mushrooms, yogurt.	1–1.4 mg 2–5 mg

Vitamin B-2 (Riboflavin)

Essential for releasing energy from foods; aids in protein synthesis.	Skin disorders, particularly around mouth. Irritated, watery, and bloodshot eyes. Brain and nervous-system problems, including personality disturbances, depression, and hysteria.	Lean meats, poultry, fish, peanuts, eggs, whole grains, dried peas and beans.	1.2–1.6 mg 2–5 mg

Vitamin B-3 (Niacin)

Crucial to breakdown of food for energy; vital for brain and nervous-system functioning. Improves circulation and lowers blood cholesterol.	Nervous irritability, headaches, insomnia, digestive disorders, swollen, sore tongue. Pellagra is the severe deficiency disease: skin disorders, diarrhea, irritability, insomnia, mental confusion.	Lean meats, poultry, fish, peanuts, eggs, whole grains, dried peas and beans.	13–18 mg	100–200 mg

Vitamin B-6 (Pyridoxine)

Helps the body break down and use fats, carbohydrates, and proteins; helps release glycogen for energy. Needed for formation of red blood cells and proper functioning of nervous tissue.	Skin disorders, cracks around the mouth, sore red tongue. Anemia, dizziness, weakness, depression, nausea, vomiting, weight loss, irritability, mental confusion, and convulsions may also result.	Whole grains, legumes, spinach, asparagus, broccoli, cauliflower, beet greens.	2–2.2 mg	2–5 mg

Appendix A: Charts and Worksheets   197

Vitamin B-12 (Cobalamin)

Works closely with folacin to manufacture DNA and RNA: necessary for proper formation of red blood cells. Helps the nervous system to function properly.	Anemia; digestive problems including indigestion, abdominal pain, constipation, diarrhea. More severe deficiencies lead to nervous-system deterioration: unsteadiness, numbness and tingling in feet, sore back, mental confusion.	Milk products, liver, kidney, fish, oysters, eggs, and nutritional yeasts.	3 mcg	Supplements not usually required.

Folacin (Folic Acid)

Essential in formation of DNA and RNA and for proper formation of red blood cells.	Common in alcoholics. Symptoms same as for B-12 (above).	Dark green leafy vegetables; liver, kidneys, wheat germ, dried peas and beans.	400 mcg	400 mcg

Pantothenic Acid

Function	Deficiency Symptoms	Sources	RDA	Supplement
Helps in metabolism of carbohydrates, proteins, and fats; important for proper functioning of adrenal glands.	Common in alcoholics. Fatigue, headaches, nausea, vomiting, sleep disturbances, abdominal cramps, muscle cramps, impaired coordination.	Yeast, liver, kidneys, milk, egg yolks, vegetables.	4–7 mg*	20–50 mg

Biotin

Function	Deficiency Symptoms	Sources	RDA	Supplement
Assists in the use of fats, carbohydrates, proteins, folic acid and pantothenic acid. Necessary for the health and maintenance of skin, hair, nerves, bone marrow, and sex glands.	Deficiency symptoms are rare, but can be caused by eating large amounts of raw eggs, which destroy biotin. Symptoms include: nausea, poor appetite, depression, muscle pains, skin problems, sleep disturbance, lack of energy.	Egg yolks (cooked), liver, whole-grain rice, brewer's yeast, dark green vegetables. Found in all animal and plant tissues.	100–200 mcg*	100–200 mcg

* No RDA has been established, but this is considered a safe and adequate dosage.

Choline

Functions	Deficiency symptoms	Sources		Dosage
A basic constituent of lecithin. Essential for the use of fats and cholesterol in the body. Helps keep nerve fibers healthy, assists in transmission of nerve impulses, and regulates liver and gallbladder function.	Deficiencies are rare. Insufficient supplies may contribute to liver, heart, and kidney disorders.	Lecithin, liver, brewer's yeast, wheat germ, egg yolks.	None established.	100–200 mg

Inositol

Functions	Deficiency symptoms	Sources		Dosage
With choline, helps dissolve fats. Necessary for cell growth and health in the intestines, eye membranes, and bone marrow.	May cause constipation, eczema, eye abnormalities, hair loss, high blood cholesterol levels.	Whole grains, lecithin, citrus fruits, brewer's yeast, liver.	None established.	100–200 mg

Pangamic Acid

Functions	Deficiency symptoms	Sources		Dosage
Helps regulate fat and sugar metabolism, stimulates glucose oxidation, promotes protein metabolism, supplies oxygen to heart, stimulates glandular and nervous systems.	A deficiency may contribute to various disorders in the heart, glandular, and nervous systems.	Whole grains, brewer's yeast, pumpkin and sesame seeds.	None established.	Unknown

PABA (Para-Amino-Benzoic Acid)

Aids in breakdown and use of proteins in body and in formation of blood cells. Can protect against sunburn and skin disturbances; may prevent skin cancer.	Not known.	Liver, brewer's yeast, yogurt, milk, eggs, whole-grain rice and cereals, whole wheat, wheat germ, molasses.	None established.	Amounts less than 30 mg are considered safe. High doses over a period of time may be toxic to liver, heart, and kidneys.

Vitamin B-17

Unknown at this time.	Not known.	Seeds of most fruits (but citrus fruits contain only small amounts).	None established.	Unknown.

Major Roles	Deficiency Symptoms	Food Sources	RDA	Safe Maintenance Doses for Alcoholics
Calcium				
Builds strong bones and teeth; maintains cell membranes; important for muscle contraction, normal heart action, nervous-system functioning, blood clotting. Involved in enzyme activity. Helps metabolize iron.	Distorted bone growth in children; softening and loss of bones in adults, with increased risk of broken bones. Retarded tooth development. Stunted growth. Cramps, spasms, heart palpitation, insomnia, nervous-system irritability.	Dried beans and peas, cheeses, milk, dark leafy vegetables, bone meal, yogurt, buttermilk, sesame seeds, sardines, nuts.	800 mg	500–1,000 mg for initial 1–3 months. Further dosages under medical supervision.
Phosphorus				
Involved in virtually all physiological chemical reactions. Builds bones and teeth, essential for release of energy from food. Essential to formation of cell membranes, enzymes, genetic material. Needed for transmission of nerve impulses and muscle contraction. Functions with calcium.	Poor mineralization of bones. Poor growth. Weakness, loss of appetite and weight.	Seeds, nuts, dried beans and peas, dried fruit, meat, poultry, fish, eggs, milk, milk products.	800 mg	Supplements not usually required.

Magnesium

Functions	Deficiency symptoms	Sources		
Builds bones. Aids in manufacture of proteins and carbohydrates and in conducting nerve impulses to muscles. Aids in regulation of acid-alkaline balances. Partner in some enzyme reactions and in energy production. Releases energy from muscle glycogen; aids in adjustment to cold.	Common in alcoholics. Muscle cramps, spasms, seizures, irregular heart beat. Sensitivity to noise, confusion, marked depression, failure to grow, pallor, weakness. Kidney damage.	Leafy green vegetables, meat, milk, nuts (especially almonds and cashews), legumes, whole grains, soybeans, seeds.	300–350 mg*	250–500 mg for initial 1–3 months. Further dosages under medical supervision.

Potassium

Functions	Deficiency symptoms	Sources		
Transmits nerve impulses; aids in muscle contraction; normalizes heart rhythm; maintains fluid and mineral balance in cells; releases energy from food.	Water retention (edema), irregular heart beat, nervous system upsets, muscular weakness, hypoglycemia, sodium imbalances.	Meats, fish, coffee, tea, most vegetables, citrus fruits, dried fruits, dried peas and beans, bananas.	1,875–5,625 mg*	Supplements not usually required.

Sodium

Function	Symptoms	Sources	Amount
Essential for normal growth; involved in mineral balance, body-fluid volume, and nerve-impulse conduction. Helps nerves and muscles function properly.	Overabundance is greater problem, but deficiency symptoms include nausea, vertigo, mental apathy, heat prostration, muscular weakness, cramps, respiratory failure.	Salted and pickled foods, salt, shellfish, cured ham, bacon, bread, crackers, most canned foods, carrots, beets, artichokes, kelp.	1,100–3,300 mg*

Sulfur

Function	Symptoms	Sources	Amount
Helps maintain oxygen balance necessary for proper brain functioning; aids liver in bile secretion; essential for healthy hair, skin, and nails.	Eczema, rashes, dermatitis, sluggishness, brittle hair and nails.	Meat, fish, soybeans, cabbage, eggs, wheat germ, dried peas and beans, peanuts, clams.	An adequate protein diet provides sufficient amount.

* These are estimated safe and adequate amounts.

Chlorine

Function	Deficiency	Sources	RDA	Supplement
Maintains and regulates balance of body fluids, electrolytes. Stimulates production of hydrochloric acid in stomach; activates enzymes in saliva.	Disturbed digestion, carbon dioxide buildup. Loss of hair and teeth.	Table salt, tomatoes, celery, kelp, olives.	1,700–5,100 mg*	Not required.

Iron

Function	Deficiency	Sources	RDA	Supplement
Essential to formation of hemoglobin (in blood) and myoglobin (in muscles), which supply oxygen to cells. An essential part of certain enzymes, thus helping to promote protein metabolism.	Anemia: fatigue, weakness, shortness of breath.	Liver (pork, calf, beef, chicken), kidneys, red meat, molasses, egg yolks, green leafy vegetables, dried fruits, dried peas and beans.	10 mg (M), 18 mg (F)	RDA is usually adequate.

Iodine

Function	Deficiency	Sources	RDA	Supplement
Assists in energy production; part of thyroid hormones; essential for normal reproduction; promotes healthy hair, nails, skin, and teeth.	Fatigue and apathy, low blood pressure, slow pulse, weight gain, lack of energy. Goiter (enlarged thyroid, with low hormone production). In newborns, cretinism (retarded growth, protruding abdomen,	Seafood, seaweed, Swiss chard, turnip greens, iodized salt, sea salt.	150 mcg	Supplements not usually required.

Copper

Functions with iron in the body's hemoglobin formation. Necessary for production of RNA: aids in development of bones, brain, nerves, connective tissue, pigment formation. Essential for utilization of vitamin C.	Anemia, abnormal development of bones and nervous tissue. Loss of hair, skin rash, heart damage.	Shrimp, most seafood, liver, kidneys, nuts, raisins, prunes, dried peas and beans, corn oil margarine.	2–3 mg*	1–3 mg

Cobalt

Essential for red blood cells; a necessary component of vitamin B-12.	Anemia, though deficiencies are rare.	Meat, kidneys, liver, milk, oysters, clams.	None established.	Not required.

* These are estimated safe and adequate amounts.

Manganese

Activates numerous enzymes; plays a role in the metabolism of carbohydrates, proteins, and fats; essential for proper functioning of nervous system, reproduction, and normal bone structure. **Needed with choline to utilize fat; necessary for utilization of some B vitamins and vitamin C.**	Deficiencies can affect glucose tolerance and may cause failure of muscle coordination, dizziness, and hearing loss.	Nuts, whole grains, green leafy vegetables, wheat germ, bran.	2.5–5.0 mg*	10–15 mg

Zinc

Found in liver, bones, skin and hair tissues, blood, pancreas, kidneys, and pituitary glands. A constituent of insulin. Essential for protein synthesis and carbohydrate metabolism. Effects transfer of carbon dioxide and maintains blood cholesterol levels. Aids in wound healing. Constituent of numerous	Retarded growth, low resistance to infection, delayed wound healing, loss of appetite, loss of fertility. A deficiency interferes with formation of RNA and DNA.	Meat, liver, poultry, eggs, milk, whole grains, nuts, green leafy vegetables, wheat germ.	15 mg	15–25 mg

Molybdenum

Constituent of certain enzymes; aids in carbohydrate and fat metabolism. Antagonist of copper.	None known in human beings. In animals: weight loss, shortened life span.
Legumes, liver, kidneys, cereal grains, yeast.	0.15–50 mg*
RDA is usually adequate.	

Selenium

Acts as an antioxidant, preventing fats from breaking down to harmful substances. Works closely with vitamin E.	Deficiency symptoms unknown in human beings. In animals: protects against liver damage and muscle degeneration. In humans may slow down aging process and protect against cancer.
Seafood, whole-grain cereals, meat, chicken, wheat germ, bran, tuna, egg yolk, milk, onions, tomatoes, broccoli.	None established.
20–50 mcg	

* These are estimated safe and adequate amounts.

Chromium

Function	Deficiency	Sources	Amount	Comment
Metabolism of glucose, integral part of some enzymes and hormones.	Abnormal sugar metabolism; may contribute to onset of diabetes in adulthood.	Meat, shellfish, cheese, whole-grain breads and cereals, brewer's yeast, dried beans, peanuts.	0.05–0.20 mg*	RDA is usually adequate.

Fluorine

Function	Deficiency	Sources	Amount	Comment
Forms strong teeth, hardens tooth enamel, maintains bone strength.	Tooth decay. In large doses, fluorine is highly poisonous.	Fish, tea, fluoridated water, most animal foods, green leafy vegetables.	1.5–4.0 mg*	Not required.

* These are estimated safe and adequate amounts.

Other Trace Elements Found in the Human Body for Which Deficiencies Have Not Been Established:

Aluminum	Helium	Rubidium
Argon	Lanthanum	Scandium
Arsenic	Lead	Silicon
Berylium	Lithium	Strontium
Boron	Mercury	Tin
Bromine	Neodymium	Titanium
Cadmium	Neon	Vanadium
Cerium	Nickel	

VITAMIN AND MINERAL LIST

Vitamin/Mineral	Natural Source	Dosage	Frequency	Reaction

EXERCISE LOG

Day	Time	Situation/Feelings	Exercise	Duration	Reactions
1					
2					
3					
4					
5					
6					
7					

HEALTH EVALUATION

Complete this form before you see your doctor, then share it with him or her.

PART I

1. My drug of choice was (check):

   ☐ Alcohol

   ☐ Cocaine

   ☐ Valium

   ☐ Amphetamines (speed)

   ☐ Heroin

   ☐ Other: _____

2. I have been addicted for:

   ☐ 2–5 years

   ☐ 5–10 years

   ☐ 10–15 years

   ☐ 15–25 years

   ☐ Other: _____

3. I have entered treatment programs _____ times.

4. I smoke (circle)   yes   no

   How much? _____

PART II

	Yes	No	Specify
1. Physical limitations	☐	☐	_____
2. Heart condition/palpitations	☐	☐	_____
3. Diabetes	☐	☐	_____
4. Hypertension	☐	☐	_____
5. Gastritis and other stomach problems	☐	☐	_____
6. Headaches	☐	☐	_____
7. Dizziness	☐	☐	_____
8. "Shakes"	☐	☐	_____
9. Hallucinations	☐	☐	_____
10. Asthma	☐	☐	_____
11. Back problems	☐	☐	_____
12. Arthritis	☐	☐	_____
13. Bursitis	☐	☐	_____
14. Muscle/joint pain	☐	☐	_____
15. Sciatica/pinched nerves	☐	☐	_____
16. Frequent colds	☐	☐	_____

Other ailments: _____

PHYSICIAN'S CHECKLIST

This is a list of the basic health information you need in order to succeed with your RRP Program. When you have your complete physical, take this list along. As your doctor examines you, fill in the blanks on your form. Your doctor will undoubtedly have other tests or exams for you to undergo, or will consider some items on the list to be unnecessary, depending on your physical condition and needs. Discuss the changes you wish to make to increase your fitness and health. Together, you can decide your health priorities.

Name: _____

Date: _____

Age: _____   Weight: _____   Height: _____

Last physical: _____

Last dental checkup: _____

Surgeries Last Five Years: _____

_____

Other Comments: _____

_____

Body temperature _____

Pulse _____

Blood Pressure _____

Vision _____

Eyes/ears/nose/throat _____

Thyroid _____

Lymph nodes—neck/armpits and groin _____

_____

Heart _____

Lungs _____

Abdomen (any unusual mass?) _____

_____

Feet and ankles (swelling?) _____

_____

Liver (enlargement or abnormalities?) _____

_____

Stool exam _____

Joints (Check range of motion and any weakness in
ligaments.) _____

_____

Muscles (Check for weakness or impairment in range of
motion.) _____

_____

Neurological condition (Are further tests necessary?) _____

_____

Blood panel _____

Liver enzyme test _____

Glucose-tolerance test _____

Chest x-ray _____

Urinalysis _____

Other _____

_____

_____

_____

LIFESTYLE INVENTORY

1. What were your excuses in the past for failing to start and/or maintain a good fitness and nutrition program?

2. What time of the day do you have the most energy?

3. How much time are you willing to devote to changing your habits?

4. When can you have time all to yourself?

5. How are you going to integrate your fitness and nutrition program with your work and family responsibilities?

6. How many days a week can you exercise? (Three is the minimum.)

7. What parts of your body do you most want to work on?

8. If you have trouble losing weight on your own, are you willing to join O.A. or another weight-loss group?

9. Do you prefer exercising alone or in a group?

DAILY INVENTORY

Use this to help gauge your daily progress. With a check, indicate whether the statement describes you, and in the space provided, feel free to elaborate on your response.

	Yes	No	Comments
1. I eat three meals a day.	☐	☐	_____
2. I crave sugar products.	☐	☐	_____
3. I eat too much.	☐	☐	_____
4. I have followed my fitness program.	☐	☐	_____
5. I use moderation in my fitness program.	☐	☐	_____
6. I feel energized at the end of the day.	☐	☐	_____
7. I do not feel tense at bed time.	☐	☐	_____
8. I do not experience ill health.	☐	☐	_____
9. I can express my spiritual self.	☐	☐	_____
10. I am aware of the stress in my life and am learning how to handle it.	☐	☐	_____
11. I am learning how to have fun.	☐	☐	_____

12. I am learning self-respect.   ☐ ☐ _____

13. I like myself.   ☐ ☐ _____

14. I allow "goofing off" periods   ☐ ☐ _____
    to relax.

15. My depressions are   ☐ ☐ _____
    diminishing.

16. I have a purpose for living.   ☐ ☐ _____

17. I recognize my creative   ☐ ☐ _____
    abilities.

18. I go to at least four A.A.   ☐ ☐ _____
    meetings a week.

Additional comments:

WRITTEN COMMITMENT

I have decided to acquire healthy living habits that will last a lifetime. I fully understand what I need to do to acquire the results I desire. Therefore, each day I will take the appropriate actions that will bring me closer to my goals.

I am aware of my biggest enemy in this process—procrastination. I will destroy this character defect by:

1. Filling out the worksheets in my notebook each day. I will also keep track of my sobriety date (last time I drank or used a chemical) and the number of days I have been clean and sober.
2. Making it a point to tell my sponsor about my progress at the end of each week.
3. Recording my weight at the beginning of each week.
4. Starting each day with a nutritious breakfast, using the breakfast selections in this book.
5. Rewarding myself after I have completed each week of faithful record keeping. (Worksheets don't have to be filled out perfectly.)

I can see my body become stronger and realize that the amount of strength I am gaining is in direct proportion to the amount of time I exercise.

I can feel my mind clearing up and am experiencing the ability to appreciate my feelings. I sense control over my responses to difficult situations. My self-confidence is returning, and with it, increased self-esteem.

I am experiencing a "spiritual awakening" through prayer and meditation. I know there is a Higher Power (which some call God), who is guiding me along life's path.

I understand that by taking action, I am developing the necessary foundation for a new healthy life in sobriety.

Signed _____

Date   _____

PERSONAL FITNESS PROFILE

	Now Date:	1 Month Date:	2 Months Date:	3 Months Date:	4 Months Date:
Resting heart rate (beats/min.)					
Recovery rate (beats/min.)					
Maximum pulse rate (beats/min.)					
Flexibility (in.)					
Sit-ups (no./min.)					
Push-ups (no./min.)					

WEEKLY EXERCISE WORKSHEET

Day/Date	Stretches	Aerobics	Strength Training	Sports/ Recreation	Comments

TRAINING DIARY

Exercise	Sets	Reps	Weight	Date	Date	Date	Date	Date

GOALS FOR HEALTH WORKSHEET

1. Check the areas you need to work on. Add others of your choice.

	Short-Term Goal	*Long-Term Goal*
☐ Improve Appearance		
☐ Lose weight		
☐ Trim inches		
☐ Firm and tone		
☐ Increase strength		
☐ Build muscles		
☐ Reduce coronary risk		
☐ Lower tension		
☐ Enjoy sports		
☐ Make new friends		
☐ Improve flexibility		
☐ Stimulate circulation		

☐ Strengthen immune system		
☐ Gain weight		
☐ Build endurance		
☐ Increase vitality		
☐ Improve stamina		
☐ Have fun		
☐ Sleep better		
☐ Learn a new sport		
☐ Quit smoking		
☐ Eat healthy foods		
☐		
☐		
☐		

2. Check whether you want to reduce or firm these body areas, and indicate what your final goals would be. Refer to your Measurement Chart from Chapter 4.

Body Area	Reduce	Firm	Goals
Shoulders	☐	☐	_____
Chest/bustline	☐	☐	_____
Upper back	☐	☐	_____
Lower back	☐	☐	_____
Upper arms	☐	☐	_____
Waistline	☐	☐	_____
Abdomen	☐	☐	_____
Hips	☐	☐	_____
Thighs	☐	☐	_____

STRESS ASSESSMENT

Place a check in the box that represents your answer.

	Yes	No
Low-back pain	☐	☐
Tension headaches	☐	☐
Migraine headaches	☐	☐
Grinding teeth	☐	☐
Acid stomach	☐	☐
Upset stomach	☐	☐
Vomiting	☐	☐
Diarrhea	☐	☐
Constipation	☐	☐
Abdominal cramps	☐	☐
Burping	☐	☐
Excess gas	☐	☐
Frequent colds	☐	☐
Tightness in chest	☐	☐
Chest pains	☐	☐

Allergies   ☐   ☐

Skin rashes   ☐   ☐

Dry mouth   ☐   ☐

Laryngitis   ☐   ☐

Shakiness   ☐   ☐

Twitches   ☐   ☐

Dizziness   ☐   ☐

Anxiety   ☐   ☐

Unrealistic fears (phobias)   ☐   ☐

Worrying   ☐   ☐

Restlessness   ☐   ☐

Depression   ☐   ☐

Sense of impending doom   ☐   ☐

Lack of concentration   ☐   ☐

Poor memory   ☐   ☐

Crying spells   ☐   ☐

Frustration   ☐   ☐

Hopelessness   ☐   ☐

Insomnia   ☐   ☐

Nightmares   ☐   ☐

Difficulty in waking up   ☐   ☐

Frequent accidents   ☐   ☐

Memory lapses   ☐   ☐

Obsessive thoughts   ☐   ☐

Loss of appetite   ☐   ☐

Overeating (excessive hunger)   ☐   ☐

Poor eating habits   ☐   ☐

Feeling of being overwhelmed by work   ☐   ☐

No time to relax   ☐   ☐

Inability to meet commitments   ☐   ☐

Isolation   ☐   ☐

Lack of sexual interest   ☐   ☐

Other symptoms: _____

_____

_____

DAILY STRESS DETECTION LOG

Carry this in your Recovery/Relapse-Prevention Program note-book during the day. When you feel stressed, fill in these blanks.

1. Time, date, day:

2. Stressful event:

3. Degree of stress felt (low, moderate, high):

4. Physical response before, during, and after:

5. Your feelings before and during a stressful event:

6. Your feelings physically and emotionally *after* a stressful event:

PERSONAL ATTITUDE INVENTORY

	Sometimes	*Always*	*Never*
1. Do I hold bad feelings toward anyone?	☐	☐	☐
2. Am I resentful for long periods of time?	☐	☐	☐
3. Do I want to get even?	☐	☐	☐
4. Do I judge others harshly?	☐	☐	☐
5. Do I judge myself harshly?	☐	☐	☐
6. Do I want to retaliate for wrongs done to me?	☐	☐	☐
7. Am I bitter about what life has done to me?	☐	☐	☐
8. Am I prejudiced toward peoples' race, religion, or social status?	☐	☐	☐
9. Do I forgive outwardly or hold in resentments?	☐	☐	☐
10. Do I love people with expectations?	☐	☐	☐
11. Do I insist things be done my way?	☐	☐	☐
12. Do I envy my neighbor?	☐	☐	☐

13. Do I blame others because of the bad luck in my life?   ☐   ☐   ☐

14. Do I blame others for my problems?   ☐   ☐   ☐

15. Do I wallow in self-pity?   ☐   ☐   ☐

16. Do I try to be cheerful?   ☐   ☐   ☐

17. Do I know my major fears?   ☐   ☐   ☐

18. Do I allow myself to make mistakes?   ☐   ☐   ☐

19. Am I living one day at a time, or do I project?   ☐   ☐   ☐

20. Do I count my blessings?   ☐   ☐   ☐

YOUR COMMITTEE'S CRITICISMS

_____

_____

_____

_____

_____

_____

_____

YOUR COMPLIMENTS AND GOOD QUALITIES

_____

_____

_____

_____

_____

_____

_____

YOUR AFFIRMATIONS

1. I believe I am a special human being.
2. I am a possibility thinker.
3. I am entitled to have abundance in my life.
4. I can handle my problems with help.
5. Today is fantastic. Something wonderful is going to happen.
6. I thank my Higher Power and myself for keeping me clean and sober.
7. I am a success.
8. I take time to appreciate nature.
9. I can change unpleasant situations.
10. I do have control over the events in my life.
11. My life is fulfilling.
12. I can let go of my anger.
13. I forgive those I am resentful toward.
14. I accept what I can't change.
15. I am strong and healthy.
16. I am a winner.

Others: _____

RRP PROGRAM REVIEW

Directions: Answer each question by choosing:

1—Always
2—Frequently
3—Sometimes
4—Never

Diet

_____ 1. I eat well-balanced meals.

_____ 2. I avoid the use of sugar.

_____ 3. I eat only at regular mealtimes.

_____ 4. I eat a piece of fruit to eliminate my sugar cravings.

_____ 5. I do not go on eating binges.

_____ 6. I chew my food thoroughly.

_____ 7. I include vitamin supplements when necessary.

_____ 8. I have eliminated caffeine.

Exercise

_____ 9. I work out three times a week for at least thirty minutes.

_____ 10. I understand how exercise can negate stress.

_____ 11. I enjoy my regular exercise routine.

_____ 12. I try to walk instead of taking rides for short distances.

_____ 13. I do daily stretches and other calisthenics routines.

_____ 14. I participate in a variety of exercise activities.

_____ 15. I have an exercise buddy.

_____ 16. I understand how to prevent sports injuries.

Health Skills

_____ 17. I have stopped smoking.

_____ 18. I have had a complete physical.

_____ 19. I have visited a dentist for a checkup.

_____ 20. I understand what conditions cause illness and take appropriate measures to avoid them.

_____ 21. I know I should never get too hungry, angry, lonely, or tired.

_____ 22. I rest when I feel tired.

_____ 23. I get at least eight hours of sleep.

Coping with Stress

_____ 24. I have learned how to just say no without feeling guilty.

_____ 25. I am able to handle the stress in my life.

_____ 26. I can let the kid out and have fun.

_____ 27. I am becoming more responsible.

_____ 28. I can express myself creatively.

_____ 29. I frequently go to A.A. meetings.

_____ 30. I have an A.A. sponsor I confide in.

Success

_____ 31. I feel accepted and loved by my fellow A.A.'ers.

_____ 32. I am clean and sober.

_____ 33. I have a spiritual direction.

_____ 34. I set realistic goals and evaluate my progress.

_____ 35. I have learned that my serenity is related to my expectations.

_____ 36. I participate in recreational pursuits in a noncompetitive environment.

_____ 37. I can ask people for help when I need it.

_____ 38. I am involved in 12-Step work (volunteer work in hospitals and institutions).

_____ 39. I am dependable.

_____ 40. I can laugh at myself and not take life so seriously.

Total Score	Results
40–50	Outstanding
51–60	Good
61–80	Fair (average)
81–120	Poor

The statements you placed a 4 next to need to be reevaluated. Try to gradually improve in these areas. Your lifetime habits cannot change overnight. Change takes time. There is no magic to transform you immediately into a stress-free, healthy, recovering person. Review your program every thirty days. The results will be impressive.

Appendix B:
Recipes

This recipe guide is to be used to complement your RRP Nutrition Program. These recipes are low in fat and are mostly sugar-free. You will find the food to be light, nutritious, and appetizing. All of these recipes take little time to prepare.

Baked Egg

½ tbsp. cooked mixed vegetables
1 egg
salt and freshly ground pepper
1 tsp. whipping cream

Put the cooked vegetables into a small baking dish. Break in one egg and sprinkle with salt and pepper. Pour the whipping cream onto the egg. Bake in a preheated moderate oven (350 degrees) for 7 minutes. Serve at once.

Serves 1

Baked Fish

---

1 6-oz. cod steak (or halibut)
3 scallions, minced
small piece of ginger root, finely chopped
grated rind of ½ lemon
lemon slices and parsley sprig

Place fish in an ovenproof dish. Sprinkle with the scallions, ginger, and lemon rind. Cover and chill for 2–3 hours.

Cover and cook in a preheated moderate oven (350 degrees) for 15 minutes or until fish is tender and flaky. Serve with parsley and lemon slices.

Serves 1

Baked Chicken

1½-lb. chicken breast
salt and freshly ground pepper
sprig of fresh tarragon
1 bay leaf
½ cup chicken stock
½ tsp. cornstarch
1 tbsp. water
2 tsp. lemon juice
8 grapes, seeded and skinned

Skin the chicken breast and sprinkle with salt and pepper. Place on a piece of foil large enough to enclose it, lay the tarragon and bay leaf on top, and fold up the foil. Bake in a preheated moderate oven (350 degrees) for about 1 hour.

Remove the chicken and keep warm. Add the juices to the chicken stock in a saucepan. Mix cornstarch with water and stir into the stock. Bring to a boil, stirring, and add the lemon juice and seasonings. When the sauce is thickened, add the grapes and continue to cook for 5 minutes. Pour the sauce over the chicken before serving.

Serves 1

Lamb Kebab

3 small tomatoes
4 quartered pieces of red or green pepper, blanched
5 oz. sliced lamb
6 pearl onions or quarters of a large onion

Thread the tomatoes, peppers, lamb, and onions alternately onto a skewer. Grill or broil for 7–8 minutes each side, turning once, until all the ingredients are cooked and tender.

Serves 1

Fruit and Seafood Salad

1 small ripe honeydew melon
1 ripe conice pear
¼ cup shelled, cooked shrimp
salt and freshly ground black pepper
2 tbsp. pine nuts, toasted
2 whole shrimp and lemon twists for garnish

Halve the melon, remove seeds, scoop out the fruit and cut into bite-sized pieces. Peel, core, and dice the pear and add to the melon; stir in the shrimp. Add the salt, pepper, and pine nuts, and spoon the mixture into the melon shells. Garnish with pine nuts, whole shrimp, and lemon.

Serves 2

Lasagna with Meat Sauce

4 lasagna noodles
8 oz. ricotta cheese
3 tbsp. grated parmesan cheese

1 cup lean ground beef
1 onion, chopped
1 8-oz. can stewed tomatoes
4 oz. tomato paste
1 bay leaf
1 tsp. oregano
salt and freshly ground black pepper
½ cup beef bouillon

For meat sauce, put the beef and onion in a saucepan and cook gently for 5 minutes, stirring occasionally. Stir in tomatoes and tomato paste; add bay leaf, oregano, salt, pepper, and bouillon. Simmer for 20 minutes.

Meanwhile, cook the lasagna noodles in boiling salted water until tender (about 5 minutes), then drain well. Put a layer of lasagna noodles in an ovenproof dish, cover with half the meat sauce and ricotta cheese, then repeat the layers, finishing with the ricotta cheese. Sprinkle the parmesan cheese on top and bake in a preheated oven (350 degrees) for 25–30 minutes, until browned and heated through.

Serves 2

Ratatouille

1 zucchini, sliced
2 tomatoes, skinned, seeded, and chopped
½ small onion, sliced
¼ small eggplant, sliced
⅔ cup tomato juice
½ clove garlic, crushed
salt and freshly ground pepper

Put all the ingredients in a saucepan and season with freshly ground pepper. Bring to a boil, then simmer, stirring occasionally, for 15–20 minutes until the vegetables are soft and the liquid reduced.

Serves 1

Trout with Almonds

1 7-oz. trout, cleaned
juice of ¼ lemon
2 tbsp. sliced almonds
watercress and lemon wedges

Sprinkle the trout with lemon juice, and place in a shallow pan. Broil for about 5–7 minutes on each side or until tender. Place the almonds in a small frying pan and heat gently until golden brown. Sprinkle over the trout and serve with lemon wedges and sprigs of watercress.

Serves 1

Tacos

¼ cup chopped lettuce
⅛ cup chopped tomatoes
2 tbsp. grated cheese
1 tbsp. chopped onion
corn tortillas

Sprinkle tortillas with lettuce, tomatoes, cheese, and onion. You can also add refried beans, sautéed ground beef, or bean sprouts.

Serves 1

Tuna Casserole

1 can (8 oz.) tuna packed in water
1 cup thinly sliced celery
2 tsp. chopped onion
1½ cups cooked whole-grain rice
½ cup walnuts
1 can (8 oz.) vichyssoise soup (cream)
¼ tsp. pepper
1 tbsp. lemon juice
3 tbsp. sugarless mayonnaise
¼ cup water
3 hard-boiled eggs, sliced

Preheat oven to 450 degrees. Combine all but last 3 ingredients in a bowl. Mix mayonnaise with water and add to tuna mixture. Slowly stir in sliced eggs. Turn mixture into lightly greased casserole and bake for 15 minutes.

Serves 4

Strawberry Yogurt

1 box strawberries, washed and sliced
2 cups plain yogurt
½ cup unsweetened apple juice
⅓ cup Grape Nuts

Puree half the strawberries, 1 cup yogurt, and apple juice in blender. Stir in remaining strawberries and Grape Nuts. Serve over, or mixed with, the rest of the yogurt.

Serves 4

Appendix C:
Reading List

The following materials were helpful in the preparation of this book. I highly recommend them to further your self-knowledge.

Addictive Drinking. Clark Vaughan. New York: Viking Press, 1982.

Alcohol Problems and Alcoholism: A Comprehensive Survey. James E. Royce. New York: Free Press, 1980.

Alcoholics Anonymous. New York: A.A. World Services, 1955.

Being Fit: A Personal Guide. Bud Getchell with Wayne Anderson. New York: John Wiley & Sons, Inc., 1982.

Body, Mind and Sugar. E. M. Abakamson, M.D., and A. Pezet. New York: Avon Books, 1977.

The Disease Concept of Alcoholism. E. M. Jellinek. Center City, MN: Hazelden Foundation, 1960.

Dr. Atkins' Nutrition Breakthrough. Robert C. Atkins, M.D. New York: William Morrow & Co., 1981.

Earl Mindell's Vitamin Bible. Earl Mindell. New York: Rawson Associates, 1979.

Eating Right to Live Sober. Katherine Ketcham and L. Ann Mueller, M.D. New York: Madrona Publishers, 1983.

The Emergent Comprehensive Concept of Alcoholism. James R. Milam. Kirkland, WA: ACA Press, 1974.

From Burnout to Balance. Dennis T. Jaffee and Cynthia D. Scott. New York: McGraw-Hill, 1984.

Health Related Physical Fitness Test Manual. Reston, VA: American Alliance for Health, Physical Education, Recreation and Dance (AAHPERD), 1980.

"High Tech" Training. Bill Dobbins. New York: Simon and Schuster, 1982.

Hypoglycemia: A Better Approach. Paavo Airola, D.D., Ph.D. Phoenix, AZ: Health Plus Publishers, 1977.

Is Alcoholism Hereditary? Donald Goodwin, M.D. New York: Oxford University Press, 1978.

Jane Brody's Nutrition Book. Jane Brody. New York: Bantam Books, 1981.

The Law of Success. Napoleon Hill. Chicago: Success Unlimited, 1969.

Let's Eat Right to Keep Fit. Adelle Davis. New York: Harcourt Brace Jovanovich, 1970.

Life After Stress. Martin Shaffer, Ph.D. New York: Plenum Press, 1982.

Low Blood Sugar and You. Carlton Fredericks and Herman Goodman. New York: Putnam, 1969.

The Low Blood Sugar Cookbook. Francyne Davis. New York: Bantam Books, 1974.

Medical Makeover. Robert M. Giller, M.D., and Kathy Matthews. New York: William Morrow & Co., 1986.

The Nautilus Book, revised edition. Ellington Oarden. Chicago: Contemporary Books, 1982.

The Nutritional Approach. Roger J. Williams. Austin, TX: University of Texas Press, 1959.

Presidential Sports Award Fitness Manual. Fit Com. Havertown, PA: Fit Com Corporation, 1983.

The Prevention of Alcoholism Through Nutrition. R. J. Williams. New York: Bantam Books, 1981.

Recipes for a Small Planet. Ellen Buchman Ewald. New York: Ballantine Books, 1973.

Stress Management: A Comprehensive Guide to Wellness. Edward Charlesworth, Ph.D., and Ronald G. Nathan, Ph.D. New York: Atheneum, 1984.

Stretching. Bob Anderson. Fullerton, CA: Anderson-World, 1975.

Twelve Steps and Twelve Traditions. Alcoholics Anonymous. New York: A.A. World Services, 1953.

Ultimate Fitness. Esquire Magazine Editors and Deborah Crocker. Reading, MA: Addison-Wesley, 1985.

Under the Influence: A Guide to the Myths and Realities of Alcoholism. James R. Milam and Katherine Ketcham. Seattle: Madrona Publishers, 1981.

Understanding Alcoholism. Christopher Smithers Foundation. New York: Scribner Book Co., 1968.

Vogue Complete Diet and Exercise. Deborah Hutton. New York: Harmony Books, 1985.

The Weider Book of Bodybuilding Tips and Routines. Joe Weider and Betty Weider. Chicago: Contemporary Books, 1982.

Weight Training for Beginners. Bill Reynolds. Chicago: Contemporary Books, 1982.

Index

Lao-Tzu, 61
Lat pulldowns, 137
Leg curls, 112–13, 137
Leg extensions, 112, 137
Leg presses, 137
Lifecycle, 136–37. *See also*
    Bicycling
Lifestyle Inventory, 76, 218
Liver, 28, 33, 63, 64–65
    dysfunction, 22
Liver enzyme test, 88
Low blood sugar. *See*
    Hypoglycemia
Lunges, 111–12
Lungs, 70, 71

Magnesium, 30, 59
Malnutrition, 22, 63
Manganese, 30
Massage, 168
Meal planning, 44, 54
Measurement Chart, 39, 40, 56,
    76, 182
Medical evaluation, 88, 138
Metabolic rate, 50, 71
Metabolism, and weight loss,
    49–50
Mineral Summary, 201–9
Minerals. *See* Supplements
Molybdenum, 30
Mood disorders, 27
Motivation, 3
Mueller, L. Ann, M.D., 60
Multivitamins, 59
Muscle soreness, and workout, 94
Muscles, 70, 71, 95
Muscular endurance, 86
Muscular Strength and Endurance
    Standards, 88

Narcotics Anonymous, 3, 66

Nautilus machines, 110
Nervous system, 63
Nicotine, 2, 49
Noradrenaline, 72
Nutrition
    as part of treatment, 4
    and alcohol and chemical abuse,
        27–29
    danger zones, 34–36
    poor, 11, 17
    proper, 3, 21
    and recovery, 13, 17
Nutrition program, 29–34
Nutritional foods, and weight loss,
    51
Nuts, 30–31

O.A. *See* Overeaters Anonymous
Oswold, Dr., 58
Overeaters Anonymous (O.A.), 19,
    48, 55

Personal Attitude Inventory,
    160–61, 233–34
Personal Fitness Profile, 80, 89,
    222
Phosphorus, 30
Physical conditioning, and weight
    loss, 15
Physical examination, 51
Physical fitness. *See* Fitness
Physician's Checklist, 76, 78,
    215–17
Potassium, 30
President's Council on Physical
    Fitness, 104
Prioritizing, 165
Professional guidance, 164
Protein, 31, 35, 42, 43, 44
Psychiatric care, 10, 12
Psychological effects of alcoholism,
    21–22